Health and Drugs Not Related

Frederick Mickel Huck

authorHOUSE

AuthorHouse™
1663 Liberty Drive
Bloomington, IN 47403
www.authorhouse.com
Phone: 1-800-839-8640

First published by AuthorHouse 12/3/2009

ISBN: 978-1-4490-5309-3 (sc)

Library of Congress Control Number: 2009912495

Printed in the United States of America
Bloomington, Indiana

This book is printed on acid-free paper.

This book is dedicated to:

ROBERT E MENZIE

INEZ A MENZIE

DONALD W HUCK

AURA V HUCK

DR EDE KOENIG

Special thanks to:

SANDRA V MOONEY

MATTHEW F MOONEY

JOHN DUNLAP

ANGIE INGERSOLL

Some Facts About Drugs

All drugs are potentially toxic and have side effects, and will often times cause more disease. The drug companies spend millions of dollars daily on TV, radio, newspaper, magazines, computer pop ups, billboards, etc in advertising. Their goal is to sell more drugs and to convince people into believing drugs are the only solution to all of humanity's problems. More than a hundred million prescriptions are written each year in the United States, due to the aggressive sales tactics that are used by large pharmaceutical companies to increase their profits.

Antibiotics have no effect on viruses. Pharmaceutical companies cannot exist without government subsidies, protection from the FDA, promotion of drugs by medical doctors and government sponsored endorsements. Drugs have not yet prevented any disease such as cancer, diabetes, weight problems, and etc in the USA. The above diseases are increasing each year, yet drugs sales are increasing.

All drugs promote and maintain disease. More than two hundred thousand people die every year of drug related problems. Last year, as well as in the not so distant past, the pharmaceutical industry claims it is interested in the cure of diseases, however without drugs sales at its present escalating volume it can only thrive on the continuation of disease. Drugs cause more problems, they suppress the symptoms and do not treat the causes.

Drugs are dangerous, many drugs are ineffective, and all drugs are chemicals. Drugs are not therefore any cure or prevention of most diseases. Often when people who are sick, they start taking more and more drugs, which ends up making them sicker.

The human body can heal itself. Historically it was very unusual to be sick, today it's considered normal to be sick and more people are sick.

Antibiotics interfere with the body's elimination process. Animal products are full of chemicals and diseases. Processed foods are also full of toxic chemicals that can lead to disease. These chemicals will suppress the immune system and they lack nutrition. Nutritional deficiencies cause an imbalance and will weaken and lower the immune system which makes you susceptible to viruses and bacteria infections; therefore your body may develop disease, pain and suffering. Drugs often times will cause more diseases.

Natural remedies are safe with almost no side effects, and are very effective. Therapies utilizing herbs and minerals work well with nature and have a long history of preventing diseases.

All drugs are unnatural, can be toxic, and do not belong in the human body.

Pesticides

All pesticides and food additives will contribute to diseases including, but not limited to, cancer. There are thousands of food chemicals in the foods we consume and we are not aware of them. A good example: there are several chemicals used to make non-nutrition foods delicious? Chemicals that are put into your body will often times never be voided from your body during your lifetime. The accumulation of chemicals over the years can cause attention deficit disorder, increase depression, stress, anxiety, learning disabilities, and much more. Science is not better than nature; food without nutrition will make you fat and your body will not perform properly.

Animals are injected with hormones, antibiotics, and irradiation. This greatly decreases nutrition. Tap drinking water has chlorine and fluoride. This will harden your arteries. Tap water is contaminated, fluoride is very toxic and dangerous. Chlorine also kills living organisms. If one desires the best calcium absorption then he should refrain from drinking carbonated drinks.

A person should know what is in shampoo, soap, cosmetics, sun screens, lotions, moisturizers, etc? The answer is chemicals! These products have toxins and chemicals and are harmful. See my setting up the pantry in my books. The products are easily available and do not cost you a lower quality of life. Stay away from any air fresheners they contain chemicals and poisons with one exception, (see my pantry list).If the human body lacks nutrition, it can not be replaced by a drug. Bad nutrition means very little nutrients will be absorbed. Taking drugs to improve nutrition will lead to more side effects In which more drugs will be prescribed and more side effects will appear.

All drugs cause an imbalance in the body. This creates more business in addition, to profits for the drug companies. Each year billions of dollars of government money is given to pharmaceutical companies, and not one tax dollar will go into natural remedy promotion. Each year almost two hundred thousand people will die from taking the proper dosage of the drugs from pharmaceutical companies. There are no deaths reported from taking natural remedies. Just remember the lack of drugs is not the cause of any disease. Chemicals in food cause the body to malfunction.

Chemicals are used to make food items look fresh, smell, and taste good, however, where is the real nutrition? Over processing food kills most nutrition and this includes spices full of chemicals. See ingredients listed on the box of item you are using. Most artificial sweeteners are chemically based. Processed food may have two or three hundred chemicals included. Vaccines, insulin, Botox, collagen, are animal based and are full of toxins and chemicals. Side effects from drugs are the fourth leading cause of death in the United States. To be healthy excludes drugs. Beware of chemicals designed as natural vitamins and herbs. The most profitable type of drug the pharmaceutical drug industry makes are cholesterol lowering drugs, high cholesterol is the number one side effect of high blood pressure drugs?

In the long run all drugs will cause the liver some damage. Drugs do not have a daily role in our lives; but are only used on very rare circumstances, after the crisis is over the drug residue needs to be removed by colon therapy.

Conclusion

It did not take me very long during the many hours of research to determine that drugs do not belong in the human body. The very high amounts of drugs taken by each person in the United States is very unrealistic. Any item or substance put in or on the body, no matter what the reason, has consequences, which are side effects.

The number one reason of why large amounts of chemicals and drugs are used and abused have been answered with this book. From your doctor , pharmacy, government drug research and the Food and Drug Administration, all are involved in this money making scheme. It can not be justified by anyone knowing the short and long-term side effects. These are crimes against humanity. Not only is this immoral, but all involved should be ashamed of themselves to cowardly make a living, under the suffering, pain, and death of others. The human body does not need or want any of these drugs.

Obviously there are exceptions: dentists, operations, or a severe accident which requires a substance for immense pain? This is only temporary. After the crisis is over a naturopathic doctor can help to get rid of the drug residue from the body. During the last ten years, the only drugs in my body was from the dentist; which was followed by a detox protocol. Otherwise there is no reason for any drug to be in your body; however prior to ten years ago, my life was the reverse. The drug problem in the USA is almost out of control, but it does not have to be for you or anyone else who wants good health;because good health and drugs are not related.

Guide 14 Days

The purpose of this fourteen day meal plan is to illustrate that starvation does not exist when following the plan. Instead of listing the fruit on a daily log everyday, I just list here approximately, what was eaten. For the last two years, I have reversed my two meals. The larger meal was consumed first and the second meal was mostly raw not cooked. Prior to eating breakfast, generally a half an hour after I wake, I drink a quart of warm water with two teaspoons of lemon juice, one tablespoon of inland sea water, and one tablespoon of silver mineral water. I consume approximately five pounds of fruit daily and the fruit varies according to the seasons of the year. The fourteen days are very similar (fruit meal) and they are three different colors of apples, twelve cherries, one nectarine, one mango, one slice of pineapple, one slice of cantaloupe, eight green grapes, one apricot, and one peach. In addition, I also eat eight raw Brazil nuts, six apricot nuts, one teaspoon of sunflower seeds, one teaspoon of pumpkin seeds, two capsules of calcium, and two capsules of magnesium. For dinner, I usually have a salad, which consists of red or green head lettuce. The salad consists of three radishes cut small, one long green onion cut small, one third of a carrot cut small, one half of avocado, and one half of celery stalk cut small. To complete the salad I add six tablespoons of lemon juice, approximately one tablespoon or more of Braggs Ammino, up to twelve ounces or more of two different kinds of hot sauce, bread, crackers, or corn tortillas.

Please do not copy or give away any material, not just because it is copyright protected material, but doing this will interfere with my program of feeding and educating the unhealthy. All book proceeds as of 2008 have gone into this program. Instead, my wish is that you do share your cooking with friends, family, and strangers.

Questions, concerns, and suggestions are welcome:
Phone   559 435 4069

14 Days of Meals

Day 1

Breakfast: Fruit

Raw nut combination

Jamaican Rice

Dinner: Salad

Garlic bread

Pasta

Dessert: Orange ball cookies

Notes: _____

_____

_____

Day 2

Breakfast: Fruit

Raw nut combination

Popcorn

Dinner: Salad

Crackers

Three pocket bean burritos

Spanish rice

Dessert: Apricot cream pie

Notes: _____

_____

_____

Day 3

Breakfast: Fruit

     Raw nut combination

     Habanera dry roasted nut mix

Dinner: Salad

     Potato and cabbage soup

     Corn bread

Dessert: Pecan Fudge

Notes: _____

     _____

     _____

Day 4

Breakfast: Fruit

Raw nut combination

Toast with almond butter

Dinner: Salad

Double baked potatoes

Crackers

Texan rice

Dessert: Cinnamon ice cream

Notes: _____

_____

_____

Day 5

Breakfast: Fruit

Raw nut combination

Cuban rice

Dinner: Salad

Lavish Tonir bread

Tamale casserole

Dessert: Licorice coconut cookies

Notes: _____

_____

_____

Day 6

Breakfast: Fruit

Raw nut combination

Toast with pear jam

Dinner: Salad

Lavish Tonir bread

Tamales

Jamaican rice

Dessert: Licorice ice cream

Notes: _____

_____

_____

Day 7

Breakfast: Fruit

Raw nut combination

Black-eyed pea rice

Dinner: Salad

Corn tortillas

Stuffed bell peppers

Dessert: Carob salt-water taffy

Notes: _____

_____

_____

Day 8

Breakfast: Fruit

Raw nut combination

Habanera rice

Dinner: Salad

Crackers

Pocket pizzas

Dessert: Walnut pie

Notes: _____

_____

_____

Day 9

Breakfast: Fruit

Raw nut combination

Oatmeal

Dinner: Two taco salads

Dessert: Coffee cake

Notes: _____

_____

_____

Day 10

Breakfast: Fruit

Raw nut combination

Bell pepper rice

Dinner: Salad, crackers

Lentils

Lemon and herb baked rice

Dessert: Orange tofu cookies

Notes: _____

_____

_____

Day 11
Breakfast: Fruit

Raw nut combination

Texan rice

Dinner: Salad

Lavish Tonir bread

Roast

Chinese rice

Dessert: Carob cup cookies

Notes: _____

_____

_____

Day 12

Breakfast: Fruit

Raw nut combination

Toast with cherry jam

Dinner: Salad

Corn bread

Pot pie

Dessert: Licorice caramel candy

Notes: _____

_____

_____

Day 13
Breakfast: Fruit

                Raw nut combination

                Cajun rice

Dinner: Salad

                Crackers

                Enchiladas

                Spanish rice

Dessert: Blueberry pie

Notes: _____

                _____

                _____

Day 14

Breakfast: Fruit

Raw nut combination with popcorn

Dinner: Salad

Lavish Tonir bread

Pocket   Beerocks

Lemon and olive rice

Dessert: Orange ice cream

Notes: _____

_____

_____

Recipe 246

ASHER NEUMILLER CAROB CHEESE CAKE

CRUST:

Make crust first. See special piecrust Recipe # 38 - Do not add any maple syrup.

Mix and add crust into 10 x 3 inch spring form pan lined with parchment paper.

FILLING:

Place in a vitamix or blender the following:

   Two cups tofu
   One cup soymilk
   Three tablespoons carob
   One tablespoon vanilla
   One and a half cups sucanant sugar
   One fourth cup whole wheat pastry flour
   Mix and pour into a pan.

Bake one hour and 15 minutes at 325 degrees.

Notes: _____
_____
_____

Recipe 247

ALLIE NEUMILLER CAROB CAKE

Place in a vitamix the following:

> One teaspoon vanilla
> One half cup Soymilk and one teaspoon soymilk
> One half cup tofu
> One cup water
> Two tablespoons carob
> One half teaspoon Biosalt
> One tablespoon roma
> One cup almond butter
> Two cups sucanant sugar

Mix and pour into a bowl with the following:

> Two cups sifted whole wheat pastry flour

Let ingredients sit at room temperature

Add one tablespoon yeast

Mix into one fourth cup finger warm water

Let sit for two hours in a warm place, dough will rise

Bake for 30 minutes or more at 350 degrees. Use toothpick test to see if baked.

Let cool. Add frosting.

FROSTING:

In a small bowl, mix the following:

> One teaspoon vanilla
> Three tablespoons carob
> Six tablespoons soymilk

Add enough sucanant sugar to make thick.

Note: Place one pound sucanant sugar into a vitamix to make a powder.

Notes: _____

_____

_____

Recipe 248

DR EDE VANILLA SUGAR CAKE

Place in a vitamix the following:

>One and a half teaspoons vanilla
>One cup Soymilk
>One half cup almond butter
>One teaspoon Biosalt
>One and one half cups sucanant sugar
>One half cup tofu

Mix and pour into a large bowl and add:

>Two and a half cups sifted whole wheat pastry flour

Let all ingredients sit at room temperature while yeast is rising.

Add one tablespoon yeast, mix into one fourth cup warm water

Let sit in a warm place for two hours

Mix, then place in a 10 x 3 inch pan or dish lined with parchment paper.

Bake 375 degrees for 25 - 30 minutes or until baked, Use toothpick test to see if baked.

When cooled, can add frosting; add one tablespoon vanilla for extra flavor.

Notes: _____

_____

_____

Recipe 249

WALNUT SQUARE COOKIES

Directions:

Place the following into a large bowl and mix:

One cup Sucanant sugar

One fourth cup tofu

One teaspoon vanilla

One fourth teaspoon Biosalt

One half cup sifted whole wheat pastry flour

One fourth cup maple syrup

One cup chopped walnuts

Mix and pour in an 8 x 8 inch glass dish lined with parchment paper, or can place on tray using cookie mat, form ingredients in an 8 x 8 inch square.

Bake 350 degrees for 25 -30 minutes

Cut into one inch squares when cool.

Notes: _____

_____

_____

Recipe 250

TARA SHABAFROOZ PECAN SQUARE COOKIES

Directions:

Place the following into a large bowl and mix:

>   One cup Sucanant sugar
>   One fourth cup tofu
>   One teaspoon vanilla
>   One fourth teaspoon Biosalt
>   One half cup sifted whole wheat pastry flour
>   One fourth cup maple syrup
>   One cup chopped pecans

Mix and pour in an 8 x 8 inch glass dish lined with parchment paper, or can place on tray using cookie mat, form ingredients in an 8 x 8 inch square.

Bake 350 degrees for 25 -30 minutes

Cut into one inch squares when cool.

Notes: _____

_____

_____

Recipe 251

ALMOND SQUARE COOKIES

Place the following into a large bowl and mix:

> One cup sucanant sugar
> One fourth cup tofu
> One teaspoon vanilla
> One fourth teaspoon Biosalt
> One half cup shifted whole wheat pastry flour
> One fourth cup maple syrup
> One cup chopped walnuts

Mix and pour in an 8 x 8 inch glass dish lined with parchment paper, or can place on tray using cookie mat, form ingredients in an 8 x 8 inches square.

Bake at 350 degrees for 25 -- 30 minutes

When cool cut into squares

Notes: _____
_____
_____

Recipe 252

MARGRET ANN MENZIE PECAN ROPE COOIKIES

Mix in a bowl the following:

> One half cup almond butter
> One eighth teaspoon Biosalt
> One cup Sucanant sugar flour
> One and a half teaspoon vanilla
> One fourth cup water
> One and a half cups sifted whole wheat pastry flour
> Two cups pecans grounded

Divide dough into 3 parts.

Roll into 12 inch ropes.

Cut each rope into 18 pieces.

Place on tray lined with parchment paper or cookie mat.

Bake 350 degrees for 15 minutes.

Notes: _____

_____

_____

Recipe 253

MASSOOD SHABAFROOZ WALNUT ROPE COOKIES

Mix in a bowl the following:

    One half cup almond butter
    One eighth teaspoonful Biosalt
    One cup sucanant sugar flour
    One and a half teaspoonfuls vanilla
    One fourth cup water
    One and a half cups sifted whole wheat pastry flour
    Two cups walnuts chopped

Divide dough into three parts.

Roll into twelve inch ropes.

Cut each rope into eighteen pieces.

Place on tray lined with parchment paper or cookie mat.

Bake 350 degrees for 15 minutes.

Notes: _____

_____

_____

Recipe 254

ALMOND ROPE COOKIES

Mix in a bowl the following:

    One half cup almond butter

    One eighth teaspoon Biosalt

    One cup sucanant sugar flour

    One and one half teaspoon vanilla

    One fourth cup water

    One and a half cups shifted whole wheat pastry flour

    Two cups almonds chopped

Divide dough into three parts, roll into twelve inch ropes, cut each rope into eighteen pieces.

Place:

On tray lined with parchment paper or cookie mat.

Bake 350 degrees for 15 minutes.

Notes: _____

                _____

                _____

Recipe 255

RHI COCONUT OATMEAL CAROB AND ROMA COOKIES

In a large bowl mix the following:

    Six cups maple syrup
    Two teaspoons Biosalt
    Three tablespoon carob
    Three tablespoons roma
    8.8 ounces coconut lite
    Four cups oatmeal flour

Let sit for two hours, especially if dough is too

Moist, form cookies on trays lined with parchment paper or cookie mat.

Bake 30 minutes at 325 degrees.

Notes: _____
                    _____
                    _____

Recipe 256

RHI COCONUT OATMEAL COOKIES

Place in a large bowl the following:

> Six cups maple syrup
> Two teaspoons Biosalt
> 8.8 ounces coconut lite
> Four cups oatmeal flour

Mix:

Let sit for two hours, or until dough is thick

Form cookies on trays lined with parchment, paper or cookie mat.

Bake 30 minutes at 325 degrees.

Notes: _____
_____
_____

Recipe 257

RHI COCONUT OATMEAL WHOLE WHEAT PASTRY FLOUR COOKIES

Mix in a large bowl the following:

Six cups maple syrup
One teaspoonful Biosalt
8.8 Ounces Coconut Lite
Four cups oatmeal flour
Five cups sifted whole wheat pastry flour.

Mix:

If batter is too thin let, sit for two hours.

Form cookies on trays lined with parchment paper or cookie mat.

Bake at 325 degrees for 25 minutes.

Notes: _____
_____
_____

Recipe 258

RHI CAROB COCONUT COOKIES

Mix in a large bowl the following:

    Six cups maple syrup

    One teaspoonful Biosalt

    Two cups oatmeal flour

    Three tablespoonfuls carob powder

    Three tablespoonfuls Roma

    Five cups sifted whole wheat pastry flour.

Mix.

Let stand, if dough is too thin, for two hours.

Form cookies on tray lined with parchment paper or cookie mat

Bake at 325 degrees for 25 minutes

Notes: _____

_____

_____

Recipe 259

RHI COCONUT COOKIE

Mix the following in a large bowl:

> Six cups maple syrup
> Five cups sifted whole wheat pastry flour
> One teaspoon Biosalt
> Two cups oatmeal flour
> Four cups coconut (whole)

Mix:

If batter is too thin, let stand for two hours.

Form on cookie trays lined with parchment paper or cookie mat.

Bake 350 degrees for 25 minutes

Mix until thick then add one half cup tofu and one fourth cup tofu, and then two tablespoons almond butter.

Mix until thick and add to pie or pastry.

Notes: _____

_____

_____

Recipe 260

RHI CAROB AND ROMA OATMEAL COOKIES

Place the following in a bowl and mix:

> Eight cups oatmeal flour
> Two teaspoonfuls vanilla
> Six cups maple syrup
> Two teaspoonfuls Biosalt
> One half cup carob
> One half cup Roma
> Four cups whole wheat pastry flour.

Mix:

Let sit for two hours if dough is too thin.

Form cookies on trays lined with parchment paper or cookie mat

Bake for 20 minutes at 325 degrees

Notes: _____

_____

_____

Recipe 261

RHI VANILLA DONUTS OR CAKE

Place in a vitamix the following:

  One half cup tofu
  One cup soy milk
  One half cup maple syrup
  One teaspoonful vanilla
  One half cup sucanant sugar
  Two cups sifted whole wheat pastry flour

Let sit at room temperature

Then add one tablespoonful yeast, mix with one fourth cup finger warm water

Mix and let sit for two hours or until dough rises

For cake, double Recipe.

Pour batter into cake pans.

Bake at 325 degrees for approximately one hour.

Check center with toothpick to see if baked.

For donuts: pour batter into donut mold.

Bake at 400 degrees for 10 minutes.

Can add frosting, when cool.

Notes: _____

_____

_____

Recipe 262

RHI CAROB BROWN CAKE

Mix in a large bowl the following:

    Three fourths cup soymilk

    One half teaspoonful Biosalt

    One third cup maple syrup

    One teaspoonful vanilla

    One third cup Sucanant sugar

    One half cup Carob

    One tablespoonful Roma

    Two thirds cup sifted whole wheat pastry flour

Let sit at room temperature;

Then add one tablespoonful yeast, mix with one fourth cup finger warm water.

Mix:

Let sit for two hours or until dough arises

Pour into cake pan.

Bake at 350 degrees for 25 minutes

Check to see if cake is done. Use toothpick test.

When cooled, can frost.

Use Recipe No. 23 Carob Glaze

Notes: _____

_____

_____

Recipe 263

RHI GOLDEN MACROONS

Mix in a large bowl the following:

> Two cups grated Carrots
> Six cups maple syrup
> One teaspoonful Biosalt
> Four cups Coconut
> Five cups sifted Whole wheat pastry flour.

Mix.

If dough is too thin, let sit for two hours or more

Form cookies on trays lined with parchment paper or cookie mat.

Bake 30 minutes at 325 degrees

Notes: _____

_____

_____

Recipe 264

RHI COFFEE MUFFINS

Place in a vitamix the following:

    Three fourths cup soymilk

    One half teaspoonful Biosalt

    Four tablespoonfuls Sucanant sugar

    One fourth cup tofu

Mix:

Pour into a large bowl and add:

    Two tablespoonfuls Roma

    One and three fourths cup sifted whole wheat pastry flour

Let sit until room temperature;

Then add one tablespoonful yeast, mix with one fourth cup finger warm water

Mix and let sit for two hours or until dough arises

Mix and pour into cup cake holders and put into muffin pans.

Bake at 400 degrees for 25 minutes

Frost when cooled.

Notes: _____

        _____

        _____

Recipe 265

RHI SPICED CUP CAKES

Place in a vitamix the following:

>   Two cups Sucanant sugar flour (grind first)
>   One cup tofu
>   One half teaspoonful Biosalt
>   Two teaspoonfuls cinnamon
>   Two cups soymilk

Then pour into a large bowl with the following:

>   Three cups sifted whole wheat pastry flour

Let sit until room temperature;

Then add one tablespoonful yeast, mix with one fourth cup finger warm water

Mix:

Place into cup cake holders, then place into muffin pans.

Bake at 375 degrees 15 minutes

Check to see if center is baked.

Frost while warm.

Notes: _____

_____

_____

Recipe 266

PEPPERMINT WALNUT FUDGE

In a pan, boil on warm for five minutes the following:

> One teaspoonful peppermint oil
> Two and a half cups sucanant sugar
> One cup maple syrup

Boil on warm for five more minutes and add two cups chopped walnuts.

Mix:

Boil on warm for five more minutes.

Add:

> One tablespoonful Roma
> One tablespoonful carob

Boil on warm for five more minutes and add two and a half cups almond Butter.

Continue to boil on warm for five more minutes and stir.

Then pour into a glass dish lined with parchment paper. (Dish size 8 X 8 inches)

Let cool. Cut into squares.

Notes: _____

_____

_____

Recipe 267

PEPPERMINT ICE CREAM

Place in a vitamix the following:

> One fourth to one half teaspoonful Peppermint oil
> One fourth teaspoonful Biosalt
> Two cups walnuts
> One brick or one pound tofu
> One tablespoonful almond butter
> One half cup soymilk
> Two cups maple syrup
> Three cups puffed corn

Blend until smooth, pour into 6 ounce cups and freeze.

Notes: _____

_____

_____

Recipe 268

CAROB AND ROMA ICE CREAM

Place in a vitamix the following:

    One half cup carob

    Two tablespoonfuls Roma

    One fourth teaspoonful Biosalt

    Two cups walnuts

    One brick or one pound tofu

    One tablespoonful almond butter

    One half cup Soymilk

    Two cups maple syrup

    Three cups puffed corn

Blend until smooth.

Pour into six ounce cups and freeze

Notes: _____

_____

_____

Recipe 269

CHERRY FUDGE

In a pan, boil on warm for 5 minutes the following:

One cup maple syrup
Two and a half cups sucanant sugar

Boil on warm for five more minutes and add:

One tablespoonful carob
One tablespoonful Roma

Boil on warm for five more minutes and add:

Two Cups chopped walnuts

Boil on warm for five more minutes and add:

One cup Cherries (dried)

Boil and mix for five more minutes and add:

Two and a half cups almond butter

Pour into a glass dish (8 x 8) lined with parchment paper.

Let cool for one to two hours.

Cut into squares and refrigerate.

Notes: _____

_____

_____

Recipe 270

CAROB ROMA PEPPERMINT ICE CREAM

Place in a vitamix or blender the following:

One forth teaspoon peppermint oil
One half cup soymilk
One Brick (or pound) tofu
One fourth teaspoon Biosalt
Two cups maple syrup
One tablespoon almond butter
Two cups walnuts
Three cups puffed corn
One half cup carob
Two tablespoons roma

Blend until smooth, pour into 6 ounce cups, and freeze.

Blend and freeze.

Notes: _____

_____

_____

Recipe 271

PEACH APRICOT PIE

See special pie crust Recipe No.38

Place in uncooked pie shell:

Two pounds cut apricots, and set aside in the refrigerator.

Place into a vitamix:

Two pounds peaches (minus pits)
One fourth teaspoon Biosalt
One cup sucanant sugar
One cup maple syrup

Then place in a pan:

Boil for One and a half hours on warm.

Then add 3 tablespoons tapioca flour

Boil another 30 minutes on warm and stir

(For a very firm filling, boil 30 more minutes extra)

Pour into a pie shell and add a crumb crust, using piecrust Recipe No. 38.

Do not add any maple syrup.

Bake 45 minutes at 350 degrees.

Notes: _____

Recipe 272

ROMA BAKED ALASKA

Place the following in a vitamix:

    One brick or one pound tofu
    One cup maple syrup
    One half cup sucanant sugar
    One fourth cup roma
    One cup almond butter

Blend until smooth

Place into baking dishes 7 x 7 inches. I use the same dishes for pot pies.

This Recipe requires four dishes.

Bake in oven 350 degrees for 20 minutes.

Let cool, can freeze extra.

Notes: _____

_____

_____

Recipe 273

RAISIN BAR COOKIES

DOUGH:

Place in a vitamix the following:

> One cup maple syrup
> One cup tofu
> One cup sucanant sugar
> One cup almond butter
> One teaspoon vanilla
> One half teaspoon Biosalt

Mix and add to a bowl with:

One half cup wheat germ

Two and a half cups sifted whole wheat pastry flour

Mix and let set for two hours.

_____

Using a rolling pin - roll out dough thin, into a 12 x 16 inch shape; this is the size of a cookie mat. Use extra whole wheat pastry flour -- dough should not stick to cookie mat. Cut rectangular length wise into thirds. Spread dried fruit down the center of each strip. Fold sides over filling to overlap. Cut one and one half inch bars and place on cookie trays, lined with parchment paper or cookie mat. Cut with plastic knife.

Bake 375 degrees for 20 minutes

_____

FILLING:

Place in a small pan the following:

>One cup chopped walnuts
>
>6 tablespoons lemon juice
>
>Two cup sucanant sugar
>
>One cup water
>
>Two tablespoons grated orange peel
>
>6 cups raisins

Heat on medium for 5 - 8 minutes or until thick.

Let cool completely.

Mixture will be thick.

Notes: _____

_____

_____

Recipe 274

FREDERICK HUCK POCKET BREAD FOLDING DIAGRAM

Pocket Bread, can be used for bean burritos, egg rolls, or

any other wrap.

Can use Tonir Lavash bread.

This is very thin bread 100% whole wheat.

Place mixture in centerfold, wrap and place on trays.

Bake 350 degrees for 10 minutes.

Notes: _____

_____

_____

Recipe 275

NOOSHIN MALEK SEE MOOSEH

Place into a small pan the following and boil for five to ten minutes or until most of the liquid is gone:

> One onion chopped
> One bell pepper chopped
> One tomato chopped
> One half cup cilantro
> Three tablespoons Braggs Ammino
> One tablespoon Biosalt
> One tablespoon chili powder
> One teaspoon garlic powder

Set aside until cool, and then pour into a large bowl with twelve ounces cooked rice, three baked potatoes (the skin removed).

Mix all ingredients together, place into wrap.

Bake 350 degrees for 10 minutes.

Recommend Recipe 274 for wrap. If using tonir lavash bread,

need two pounds, makes twenty items.

Notes: _____

_____

_____

Recipe 276

ZOHREH   EHSANI BLUEBERRY ICE CREAM

Place in a vitamix all of the following:

One fourth teaspoon Biosalt
One half cup soymilk
Two cups walnuts
One brick or one pound tofu
Three cups puffed corn or puffed rice
One cup blueberries
One tablespoon almond butter
Two cup maple syrup

Blend until smooth. Place in six ounce cups and freeze.

Notes: _____

_____

_____

Recipe 277

POCKET PIZZA ONE

See Recipe 274 for wrap and bake information.

Place into a vitamix twenty tomatoes. Do not add any water. Then pour into a large

Pan with the following:

    Three tablespoons oregano
    Three tablespoons thyme
    One tablespoon almond butter
    One teaspoon maple syrup
    Two teaspoons Biosalt
    Three teaspoons basil
    Three teaspoons parsley
    Four cloves garlic cut small
    Two onions chopped
    One can olives, cut each into half.

Continue to boil two hours or more, until sauce is thick. Let sauce cool. Place three cooked potatoes (minus skins) into sauce pan and mash and stir into mixture.

Wrap and place mixture and fold. Place on trays.

Bake 350 degrees for 10 minutes.

Let cool - freeze extra. Makes 24 units

Notes: _____

                _____

                _____

Recipe 278

RAISIN CREAM PIE

Wash - clean five cups raisins, set aside for one hour, and let water drain from raisins.

Then place raisins into vitamix with the following:

> One cup maple syrup
> One cup Sucanant Sugar
> One tablespoon cinnamon
> One fourth teaspoon Biosalt
> One apple (remove core only)

Pour mixture into a large pan. Boil for one half hour on warm, or until mixture is very thick. Then add to pie shell and put top crust and press into pie - do not add any maple syrup. This is a crumb crust.

See special piecrust Recipe # 38

Bake in oven 350 degrees for 45 minutes.

Let cool and serve. Freeze extra.

Helpful hint: enough filling for two pies

Notes: _____

_____

_____

Recipe 279

DR. EDE KOENIG BEEROCK

In a pan boil the following for five to ten minutes or until water is gone:

    Five sticks celery cut small

    Ten cloves garlic cut small

    One fourth a purple cabbage cut small

    One half cup cilantro cut small

    One purple onion cut small

    Two long green onions cut small

    One teaspoon Biosalt

    One tablespoon dill

    One tablespoon cumin

    Two tablespoons Braggs Ammino

    One teaspoon Savory

Then place into pan three cooked potatoes (skins removed) mash into mixture.

See Recipe 274 for wrap and bake information. Place on trays.

Bake 350 degrees for 10 minutes.

Let cool- Freeze extra.

Notes: _____

_____

_____

Recipe 280

DATE CREAM PIE

Wash - clean five cups dates. Set aside for one hour, let water drain from

Dates. Then place into vitamix with the following:

One cup Maple Syrup
One cup Sucanant Sugar
One Apple (remove core only)
One fourth teaspoon Biosalt

Then pour into a large pan and boil on low for one half hour. Then add to pie shell and put top crust, and press into pie - do not add any maple syrup this is a crumb crust.

See special piecrust Recipe # 38

Bake 350 degrees for 45 minutes.

Let cool and cut. Can freeze extra

Notes: _____

_____

_____

Recipe 281

POCKET RAISIN PASTRY

Wash - clean five cups raisins and then set aside for one hour and let water drain. Then place raisins in vitamix with the following:

> One cup sucanant sugar
> One cup maple syrup
> One tablespoon cinnamon
> One fourth teaspoon Biosalt
> One apple (remove core only)

Pour into a large pan and boil for one half hour on low and until mixture is very thick.

Let cool, place into wrap - see Recipe # 274.

Place on trays. Bake 10 minutes at 350 degrees.

Makes 20 units

Notes: _____
_____
_____

Recipe 282

POCKET PIZZA 3

See Recipe 274 for wrap and bake information.

Place into a vitamix twenty tomatoes. Do not add any water. Then pour into a large

Pan with the following:

> One half cup almond butter
> Three tablespoons oregano
> One teaspoon maple syrup
> Two teaspoons marjoram
> Two teaspoons Biosalt
> Four cloves garlic cut small
> One onion cut small
> One can olives cut each into one half.

Boil on low for two hours or more. Sauce must be very thick, let sauce cool. Then place three cooked potatoes (remove skins) into saucepan and mash and stir into mixture.

Wrap and place mixture and fold. Place on trays.

Bake 350 degrees for 10 minutes.

Let cool - freeze extra. Makes 24 units

Notes: _____

_____

_____

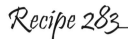*Recipe 283*

POCKET PIZZA 4

See Recipe 274 for wrap and bake information.

Place into a vitamix twenty tomatoes. Do not add any water. Then pour into a large

Pan with the following:

> One teaspoon maple syrup
> Two teaspoons cumin
> Two teaspoons dill
> Two teaspoons Biosalt
> One teaspoon marjoram
> Four teaspoons paprika
> Three tablespoons oregano
> Four cloves garlic cut small
> One onion cut small
> One can olives cut each into one half
> Four Green Peppers chopped small

Boil on low for two hours or more. Sauce must be very thick. Let sauce cool. Then place three cooked potatoes (remove skins) into saucepan and mash and stir into mixture.

Wrap and place mixture and fold. Place on trays.

Bake 350 degrees for 10 minutes.

Let cool - freeze extra. Makes 24 units.

Notes: _____

_____

_____

Recipe 284

POCKET PIZZA 2

See Recipe 274 for wrap and bake information.

Place into a vitamix twenty tomatoes. Do not add any water. Then pour into a large Pan with the following:

Three tablespoons oregano
Four tablespoon almond butter
One teaspoon maple syrup
One teaspoon Biosalt
One bell pepper cut small
Four cloves garlic cut small
One onion cut small
One can olives cut each into one half.

Boil on low for two hours or more. Sauce must be very thick. Let sauce cool. Then place three cooked potatoes (remove skins) into saucepan and mash and stir into mixture.

Wrap and place mixture and fold. Place on trays.

Bake 350 degrees for 10 minutes.

Let cool - freeze extra. Makes 24 units

Notes: _____
_____
_____

Recipe 285

POCKET DATE PASTRY

Wash - clean five cups dates and then set aside for one hour and let water drain. Then place dates in vitamix with the following:

One cup sucanant sugar
One cup maple syrup
One fourth teaspoon Biosalt
One apple (remove core only)

Pour into a large pan and boil for one half hour on low and until mixture is very thick.

Let cool, place into wrap - see Recipe # 274.

Place on trays. Bake 10 minutes at 350 degrees.

Makes 20 units.

Notes: _____

_____

_____

Recipe 286

POCKET PLUM PASTRY

Wash - clean five cups plums (remove seeds) and then set aside for one hour and let water drain. Then place plums in vitamix with the following:

    One cup sucanant sugar
    One cup maple syrup
    One fourth teaspoon Biosalt
    One apple (remove core only)

Pour into a large pan and boil for one hour on low and until mixture is very thick.

Let cool, place into wrap - see Recipe # 274.

Place on trays. Bake 10 minutes at 350 degrees.

Makes 20 units

Notes: _____
_____
_____

Recipe 287

PLUM CREAM PIE

For piecrust: See piecrust Recipe # 38

Place into vitamix the following:

    Five pounds plums (remove pits)

Do not add any water, and add the following:

    One cup sucanant sugar
    One cup maple syrup
    One apple (remove core only)
    One fourth teaspoon Biosalt

Pour mixture into large pan and boil on warm for one hour or more or until thick.

Pour into pie shell, place top crust -- do not add any maple syrup.

This is a crumb crust. Cover pie and press into pie.

Bake 350 degrees for 45 minutes.

Let cool -- and cut.

Freeze extra.

Helpful hint: enough for two pies

Notes: _____

_____

_____

Recipe 288

POCKET CAROB PASTRY

Place in a vitamix the following:

    One brick or one pound tofu
    One cup maple syrup
    One half cup sucanant sugar
    One half cup carob
    One cup almond Butter

Place into wrap -- see Recipe 274 for folding and bake information...

Place on trays.

Bake for 10 minutes at 350 degrees.

Let cool. Freeze extra.

Helpful Hints: The night before make, sure you have all the ingredients, and utensils set-up, this cuts down on your preparation time.

Notes: _____

               _____

               _____

Recipe 289

POCKET ROMA PASTRY

Place in a vitamix the following:

> One brick or one pound tofu
> One cup maple syrup
> One half cup sucanant sugar
> One half cup Roma
> One cup almond butter

Place into wrap -- see Recipe 274 for folding and bake information...

Place on trays.

Bake for 10 minutes at 350 degrees.

Let cool. Freeze extra.

Helpful Hints:

The night before make sure, you have all the ingredients and set up all your utensils, this will save time.

Notes: _____

_____

_____

Recipe 290

POCKET WALNUT PASTRY

Place the following in a large bowl and mix:

Two cups sucanant sugar
One cup tofu
Two teaspoon vanilla
One cup almond butter

Then add four cups chopped Walnuts.

Mix:

See Recipe 274 for warp and folding information...

Place the above mixture into wrap. Place on trays.

Bake for 10 minutes at 350 degrees.

Let cool. Freeze extra

Notes: _____

_____

_____

Recipe 291

POCKET APRICOT PASTRY

Wash - clean five cups apricots (remove seeds) and then set aside for one hour and let water drain. Then place apricots in vitamix with the following:

>   One cup sucanant sugar
>   One cup maple syrup
>   One fourth teaspoon Biosalt
>   One apple (remove core only)

Pour into a large pan and boil for one hour on low and until mixture is very thick.

Let cool, place into wrap - see Recipe # 274.

Place on trays. Bake 10 minutes at 350 degrees.

Makes 20 units.

Notes: _____

_____

_____

Recipe 292

POCKET CHERRY PASTRY

Wash - clean five cups cherries (remove seeds) and then set aside for one hour and let water drain. Then place cherries in vitamix with the following:

   One cup sucanant sugar
   One cup maple syrup
   One fourth teaspoon Biosalt
   One apple (remove core only)

Pour into a large pan and boil for one hour on low and until mixture is very thick.

Let cool, place into wrap - see Recipe # 274.

Place on trays. Bake 10 minutes at 350 degrees.

Makes 20 units

Notes: _____
_____
_____

Recipe 293

POCKET PEACH PASTRY

Wash - clean five cups peaches (remove pits only) and then set aside for one hour and let water drain. Then place cherries in vitamix with the following:

> One cup sucanant sugar
> One cup maple syrup
> One tablespoon cinnamon
> One fourth teaspoon Biosalt
> One apple (remove core only)

Pour into a large pan and boil for one hour on low and until mixture is very thick.

Let cool, place into wrap - see Recipe # 274.

Place on trays. Bake 10 minutes at 350 degrees.

Makes 20 units.

Notes: _____
_____
_____

Recipe 294

POCKET PINEAPPLE - LEMON PASTRY

Place One can pineapple (drain juice) in vitamix with the following:

   Six tablespoons lemon rind
   One brick or one pound tofu
   One cup sucanant sugar
   One cup maple syrup
   One fourth teaspoon Biosalt
   One apple (remove core only)

Pour into a large pan and boil for one hour on low and until mixture is very thick.

Let cool, place into wrap - see Recipe # 274.

Place on trays. Bake 10 minutes at 350 degrees.

Makes 20 units

Notes: _____
    _____
    _____

Recipe 295

POCKET PUMPKIN PASTRY

Place in a vitamix one can 100% Pumpkin and add:

> One fourth teaspoon allspice
>
> One teaspoon Biosalt
>
> One cup maple syrup
>
> One tablespoon vanilla
>
> One half cup cashews - cleaned
>
> One half cup sucanant sugar
>
> One apple (remove core only)
>
> Three fourths teaspoon cinnamon

Mix.

Then pour into a large pan. Then boil for one half hour on low or until sauce is thick.

Let cool, and for wrap and bake information see Recipe 274.

Place on trays.

Bake for 10 minutes at 350 degrees.

Let cool. Freeze extra.

Notes: _____

_____

_____

Recipe 296

POCKET APPLE PASTRY

Place in a vitamix five pounds apples (with cores removed) and add:

    One fourth teaspoon Biosalt
    One cup maple syrup
    One teaspoon Vanilla
    One cup sucanant sugar
    One apple (remove core only)
    One teaspoon cinnamon

Mix.

Then pour into a large pan. Then boil for one hour on low or until sauce is thick.

Let cool

For wrap and bake information see Recipe 274.

Place on trays.

Bake for 10 minutes at 350 degrees.

Let cool. Freeze extra.

Helpful Hints:

The night before make sure, you have all the ingredients and set up all your utensils, this will save time

Notes: _____

_____

_____

Recipe 297

POCKET EGG ROLLS

For wrap, see Recipe # 274, for wrap and folding information:

In a large pan, place the following:

Six tablespoon Braggs Ammino
One tablespoon Biosalt
Twelve radishes (shredded)
Four carrots (shredded)
Two bell peppers (shredded)
Two onions cut small
Four cups celery cut small
Eight cloves garlic cut small
Four cups cabbage cut small

Boil for 5 minutes and stir, and then add one pound bean sprouts. Then mix and continue to stir for three more minutes. Let cool and drain all juice. Wrap and place on trays.

Bake 450 degrees for 10 minutes.

Let cool. Can freeze extra

Notes: _____

_____

_____

Recipe 298

POCKET BEAN BURRITO

For wrap see Recipe 274 - for fold and wrap information.

Can use any bean Recipe: such as # 11, # 100, # 132, # 147, and # 155

Directions:

When beans are cooked, mash, then let cool and place into wrap. Place on trays

And bake at 350 degrees for 10 minutes.

Let Cool.

Freeze extra.

Helpful Hints:

The night before make sure, you have all the ingredients and set up all your utensils, this will save time.

Notes: _____

_____

_____

Recipe 299

APRICOT CREAM PIE

For piecrust: See piecrust Recipe # 38

Place into vitamix the following:

> Five pounds apricots (remove pits)
> Do not add any water, and add the following:
> One cup sucanant sugar
> One cup maple syrup
> One apple (remove core only)
> One fourth teaspoon Biosalt

Pour mixture into large pan and boil for one hour or more on warm or until thick.

Pour into pie shell, place top crust -- do not add any maple syrup.

This is a crumb crust. Cover pie and press into pie.

Bake 350 degrees for 45 minutes.

Let cool -- and cut.

Freeze extra.

Helpful hint: enough filling for two pies

Notes: _____

_____

_____

Recipe 300

VERA WALDSCHMIDT CHERRY CREAM PIE

For piecrust Recipe see # 38

Place into vitamix 5 pounds Cherries (remove pits). Do not add any water and add the Following ingredients:

    One cup maple syrup
    One cup sucanant sugar
    One apple (remove core)
    One fourth teaspoon Biosalt

Directions:

Pour mixture into large pan and boil for one hour or more on warm or until thick.

Pour mixture into pie shell. Then place top crust - do not add any maple syrup.

This is a crumb crust, cover piecrust and press into pie.

Bake at 350 degrees for 45 minutes.

Let cool. Can freeze extra.

Helpful hint:

The night before make sure, you have all the ingredients and set up all your utensils, this will save time

Enough filling for two pies

Notes: _____

_____

_____

Recipe 301

PEACH CREAM PIE

For piecrust: See piecrust Recipe # 38

Place into vitamix the following:

Five pounds peaches (remove pits)
Do not add any water, and add the following:
One cup sucanant sugar
One cup maple syrup
One apple (remove core only)
One fourth teaspoon Biosalt

Pour mixture into large pan and boil for One hour or more on warm or until thick.

Pour into pie shell, place top crust -- do not add any maple syrup.

This is a crumb crust. Cover pie and press into pie.

Bake 350 degrees for 45 minutes.

Let cool -- and cut.

Freeze extra.

Helpful Hints: this is enough filling for two pies

Notes: _____

_____

_____

Recipe 302

APPLE CREAM PIE

For piecrust: See piecrust Recipe # 38

Place into vitamix the following:

> Five pounds apples (remove cores only)
> Do not add any water, and add the following:
> One cup sucanant sugar
> One cup maple syrup
> One fourth teaspoon Biosalt

Pour mixture into large pan and boil for one hour or more on warm or until thick.

Pour into pie shell, place top crust -- do not add any maple syrup.

This is a crumb crust. Cover pie and press into pie.

Bake 350 degrees for 45 minutes.

Let cool -- and cut.

Freeze extra

Notes: _____

_____

_____

Recipe 303

TAHEREH TAHERIAN HAVANERO HOT SAUCE

Place the following in a vitamix:

 15 - 25 habanera peppers
 Two tablespoonfuls garlic powder
 One cup maple syrup
 One onion
 One cup lemon juice
 One half cup cilantro
 Two tablespoonfuls Biosalt
 Two teaspoonfuls cumin
 26 cups or 26 tomatoes
 Four to six cups water

Blend and pour into large pan, and boil for two hours on low.

When cooled, place in jars and freeze extra

Notes: _____
_____
_____

Recipe 304

SHAHNAZ SHAINEE HOT & SPICY PINTO BEANS

The night before soak 5 cups pinto beans, with enough water to cover 3 - 4 inches above the beans.

The next day boil 10 minutes and pour out water -- change water and add the following:

Two onions chopped
One half cup cilantro
Two tablespoonfuls Braggs Ammino
Four cloves garlic cut small
One tablespoonful Biosalt
Three bell peppers cut small
Four tomatoes cut small
Four tablespoonfuls cayenne pepper
Two tablespoonfuls dill
Two tablespoonfuls cumin
Two tablespoonfuls chili powder
One raw clean potato

(After beans are cooked, throw potato away)

Continue to boil on low until cooked approximately one and half to two hours.

Notes: _____

_____

_____

Recipe 305

PAYAM   MALEK ZADEH CAROB WHEAT COOKIES

In a large bowl mix all the following:

> Eight cups maple syrup
> One half cup carob powder
> One half cup Roma
> Eight teaspoonfuls almond butter
> Two teaspoonfuls vanilla
> Two teaspoonfuls Biosalt
> Twelve cups whole wheat pastry flour sifted

Mix and form cookies on cookie tray lined with parchment paper, or a cookie mat.

Bake 325 degrees for 25 - 30 minutes

Notes: _____

_____

_____

Recipe 306

RAISIN ICE CREAM

Place in a vitamix or blender the following:

Two cups clean raisins. Wash and let water drain for one hour.
One brick or one pound tofu
One half cup soymilk
One tablespoonful almond butter
Two cups maple syrup
Three cups puffed corn or puffed rice
One fourth teaspoonful Biosalt
Two cups walnuts

Blend until smooth, pour into 6 ounce cups and freeze

Notes: _____
_____
_____

Recipe 307

TOMATO CASSEROLE

Crust:

Place the following in a vitamix:

>   One fourth teaspoonful Biosalt
>   One cup oatmeal
>   One fourth cup coconut
>   One cup almonds

Mix and pour into glass pie dish and add four tablespoonfuls water.

Mix and form into pie crust.

Bake 10 minutes at 375 degrees. Set aside.

Filling:

Place into pie shell thin - sliced tomatoes, arrange to overlap.

Next in a bowl, place one can olives cut each into small pieces, and add and mix:

>   Two tablespoonfuls Braggs Ammino
>   One tablespoonful thyme
>   One tablespoon basil
>   Two tablespoonfuls lemon juice
>   One half teaspoonful cumin

Then add one half of this mixture into pie shell and spread, and add another layer very thin sliced tomatoes overlapping. This should fill up the pie shell. Then place the rest of olive mixture on top of tomatoes,

Bake 20 minutes at 375 degrees.

May need 6 - 8 tomatoes if using Roma tomatoes

Notes: _____

_____

_____

Recipe 308

RAISIN FACE COOKIE

FILLING:

Wash two and a half cups raisins and set aside. - Let water drain for one hour.

Then place into vitamix with following:

> One half cup maple syrup
> One half cup sucanant sugar
> One teaspoon cinnamon
> One fourth teaspoon Biosalt
> One apple (remove core only)

Mix and place into a pan and boil on low for one half hour or until very thick.

Stir occasionally.

DOUGH:

Place into a vitamix the following:

> One half teaspoon vanilla
> One and one half cups almond butter
> One teaspoon rosewater or can use water
> One half teaspoon Biosalt
> One cup maple syrup

Mix and add to a bowl with two cups sifted whole wheat pastry flour.

Let set until firm. May add more whole wheat pastry flour when needed.

Roll into balls and press into round cookie cutter, (2 X 2 inches) Press into cookie cutter, cookie should look like a small pie.

Place on tray lined with parchment paper or cookie mat.

Bake 5 minutes at 375 degrees.

Then place filling on top of cookies and return to oven for 5 more minutes.

This Recipe requires two trays.

Notes: _____

_____

_____

Recipe 309

DATE FACE COOKIE

FILLING:

Wash two and a half cups dates (remove pits) and set aside. - Let water drain for one hour.

Then place into vitamix with following:

> One half cup maple syrup
> One half cup sucanant sugar
> One fourth teaspoon Biosalt
> One apple (remove core only)

Mix and place into a pan and boil on low for one half hour or until very thick.

Stir occasionally.

DOUGH:

Place into a vitamix the following:

> One half teaspoon vanilla
> One and one half cups almond butter
> One teaspoon rosewater or can use water
> One half teaspoon Biosalt
> One cup maple syrup

Mix and add to a bowl with two cups sifted whole wheat pastry flour.

Let set until firm. May add more whole wheat pastry flour when needed.

Roll into balls and press into round cookie cutter, (2 X 2 inches) Press into cookie cutter, cookie should look like a small pie.

Place on tray lined with parchment paper or cookie mat.

Bake 5 minutes at 375 degrees.

Then place filling on top of cookies and return to oven for 5 more minutes.

This Recipe requires two trays.

Notes: _____

_____

_____

Recipe 310

PINEAPPLE COCONUT SQUARES

Place in a vitamix the following:

  Two cups sucanant sugar
  One half cup almond butter
  One half cup tofu
  One fourth teaspoon vanilla
  One can pineapple (drain juice)

Mix and pour into large bowl with:

  One cup coconut
  Three fourths cup sifted whole wheat pastry flour

Mix and pour into a cake pan (9 x 9 inches) lined with parchment paper.

Bake 350 degrees for 25 - 30 minutes.

Use the toothpick test to see if center is baked.

When cool cut into squares.

Notes: _____

_____

_____

Recipe 311 _____

ORANGE PINEAPPLE ICE CREAM

Place in a vitamix the following:

> One fourth teaspoon Biosalt
> Two cups walnuts
> One brick or one pound tofu
> One half cup soymilk
> One tablespoon almond butter
> Two cups maple syrup
> Three cups puffed rice or puffed corn
> 3 to 6 tablespoons orange rind
> One cup pineapple juice

Blend until smooth.

Pour into 6 ounce cups and freeze

Notes: _____

_____

_____

Recipe 312

LEMON PINEAPPLE ICE CREAM

Place in a vitamix the following:

    One fourth teaspoon Biosalt

    Two cups walnuts

    One Brick or one pound tofu

    One half cup soymilk

    One tablespoon almond butter

    Two cups maple syrup

    Three cups puffed rice or puffed corn

    3 to 6 tablespoons lemon rind

    One cup pineapple juice

Blend until smooth.

Pour into 6 ounce cups and freeze

Notes: _____

_____

_____

Recipe 313 ——————————————

ROMA FACE COOKIE

FILLING:

Place in a vitamix the following:

> One brick or one pound tofu
> One cup maple syrup
> One half cup sucanant sugar
> One half cup Roma
> One cup almond butter

Pour in a small bowl and set aside.

DOUGH:

Place into a vitamix the following:

> One half teaspoon vanilla
> One and a half cups almond butter
> One half teaspoon Biosalt
> One teaspoon rosewater or water
> One cup maple syrup

Mix and add in another bowl, with Two cups sifted whole wheat pastry flour.

May add more when needed

Roll into balls and press into round cookie cutter (2 X 2 inches). Cookies should look like a small pie.

Place on trays lined with parchment paper or a cookie mat, and put into oven.

Bake 5 minutes at 375 degrees.

Then place filling on top cookie and return to oven for 5 more minutes.

This Recipe requires two trays

Notes: _____

_____

_____

Recipe 314

CAROB FACE COOKIE

FILLING:

Place in a vitamix the following:

   One brick or one pound tofu
   One cup maple syrup
   One half cup sucanant sugar
   One half cup carob
   One cup almond butter

Pour in a small bowl and set aside.

DOUGH:

Place into a vitamix the following:

   One half teaspoon vanilla
   One and a half cups almond butter
   One half teaspoon Biosalt
   One teaspoon rosewater or water
   One cup maple syrup

Mix and add in another bowl, with two cups sifted whole wheat pastry flour.

May add more when needed.

Roll into balls and press into round cookie cutter (2 X 2 inches). Cookies should look like a small pie.

Place on trays lined with parchment paper or a cookie mat, and put into oven.

Bake 5 minutes at 375 degrees.

Then place filling on top cookie and return to oven for 5 more minutes.

This Recipe requires two trays

Notes: _____

_____

_____

Recipe 315

PUMPKIN FACE COOKIE

FILLING:

Place in a vitamix the following:

> One can 100% pumpkin
> One fourth teaspoon allspice
> Three fourths teaspoon cinnamon
> One cup maple syrup
> One fourth teaspoon Biosalt
> One half cup sucanant sugar
> One teaspoon vanilla
> One apple (remove core only)

Then place in a pan and boil on low for one half hour or until thick.

DOUGH:

Place into a vitamix the following:

> One half teaspoon vanilla
> One and a half cups almond butter
> One half teaspoon Biosalt
> One teaspoon rosewater or water
> One cup maple syrup

Mix and add in another bowl, with two cups sifted whole wheat pastry flour.

May add more when needed.

Roll into balls and press into round cookie cutter (2 X 2 inches). Cookies should look like a small pie.

Place on trays lined with parchment paper or a cookie mat, and put into oven.

Bake 5 minutes at 375 degrees.

Then place filling on top cookie and return to oven for 5 more minutes.

This Recipe requires two trays

Notes: _____

_____

_____

Recipe 316

PINEAPPLE FACE COOKIE

FILLING:

Place in a vitamix the following:

One 20 ounce can pineapple (drain juice) Do not add any water

Add:

One cup maple syrup
One fourth teaspoon Biosalt
One cup sucanant sugar
One apple (remove core only)

Mix:

Boil on low for one hour or more until mixture is thick.

DOUGH:

Place into a vitamix the following:

One half teaspoon vanilla
One and a half cups almond butter
One half teaspoon Biosalt
One teaspoon rosewater or water
One cup maple syrup

Mix:

Add in another bowl, with two cups sifted whole wheat pastry flour.

May add more when needed.

Roll into balls and press into round cookie cutter (2 X 2 inches). Cookies should look like a small pie.

Place on trays lined with parchment paper or a cookie mat, and put into oven.

Bake 5 minutes at 375 degrees.

Then place filling on top cookie and return to oven for 5 more minutes.

This Recipe requires two trays

Notes: _____

_____

_____

Recipe 317

APPLE   FACE COOKIE

FILLING:

Place in a vitamix the following:

Two and a half pounds apples (remove core only) Do not add any water

And add

One cup maple syrup
One fourth teaspoon Biosalt
One cup sucanant sugar
One apple (remove core only)

Mix:

Boil on low for one hour or more until mixture is thick.

DOUGH:

Place into a vitamix the following:

One half teaspoon vanilla
One and a half cups almond butter
One half teaspoon Biosalt
One teaspoon rosewater or water
One cup maple syrup

Mix:

Add in another bowl, with two cups sifted whole wheat pastry flour.

May add more when needed.

Roll into balls and press into round cookie cutter (2 X 2 inches). Cookies should look like a small pie.

Place on trays lined with parchment paper or a cookie mat, and put into oven.

Bake 5 minutes at 375 degrees.

Then place filling on top cookie and return to oven for 5 more minutes.

This Recipe requires two trays

Notes: _____

_____

_____

Recipe 318

PEACH FACE COOKIE

FILLING:

Place in a vitamix the following:

   Two and a half pounds peaches (remove pits) do not add any water

And add

   One cup maple syrup
   One fourth teaspoon Biosalt
   One cup sucanant sugar
   One apple (remove core only)

Mix and boil on low for one hour or more until mixture is thick.

DOUGH:

Place into a vitamix the following:

   One half teaspoon vanilla
   One and a half cups almond butter
   One half teaspoon Biosalt
   One teaspoon rosewater or water
   One cup maple syrup

Mix:

Add in another bowl, with two cups sifted whole wheat pastry flour.

May add more when needed.

Roll into balls and press into round cookie cutter (2 X 2 inches). Cookies should look like a small pie.

Place on trays lined with parchment paper or a cookie mat, and put into oven.

Bake 5 minutes at 375 degrees.

Then place filling on top cookie and return to oven for 5 more minutes.

This Recipe requires two trays

Notes: _____

_____

_____

Recipe 319

APRICOT FACE COOKIE

FILLING:

Place in a vitamix the following:

Two and a half pounds apricots (remove pits) Do not add any water

Add

One cup maple syrup
One fourth teaspoon Biosalt
One cup sucanant sugar
One apple (remove core only)

Mix;

Boil on low for one hour or more until mixture is thick.

DOUGH:

Place into a vitamix the following:

One half teaspoon vanilla
One and a half cups almond butter
One half teaspoon Biosalt
One teaspoon rosewater or water
One cup maple syrup

Mix and add in another bowl, with two cups sifted whole wheat pastry flour.

May add more when needed.

Roll into balls and press into round cookie cutter (2 X 2 inches). Cookies should look like a small pie.

Place on trays lined with parchment paper or a cookie mat, and put into oven.

Bake 5 minutes at 375 degrees.

Then place filling on top cookie   and return to oven for 5 more minutes.

This Recipe requires two trays.

Notes: _____

_____

_____

Recipe 320

PLUM FACE COOKIE

FILLING:

Place in a vitamix the following:

    Two and a half pounds plums (remove pits) Do not add any water

Add

    One cup maple syrup
    One fourth teaspoon Biosalt
    One cup sucanant sugar
    One apple (remove core only)

Mix and boil on low for one hour or more until mixture is thick.

DOUGH:

Place into a vitamix the following:

    One half teaspoon vanilla
    One and a half cups almond butter
    One half teaspoon Biosalt
    One teaspoon rosewater or water
    One cup maple syrup

Mix and add in another bowl, with two cups sifted whole wheat pastry flour.

May add more when needed.

Roll into balls and press into round cookie cutter (2 X 2 inches). Cookies should look like a small pie.

Place on trays lined with parchment paper or a cookie mat, and put into oven.

Bake 5 minutes at 375 degrees.

Then place filling on top cookie   and return to oven for 5 more minutes.

This Recipe requires two trays

Notes: _____

_____

_____

Recipe 321 _____

CHERRY   FACE COOKIE

FILLING:

Place in a vitamix the following:

   Two and a half pounds cherries (remove pits) Do not add any water

Add

   One cup maple syrup
   One teaspoon Biosalt
   One cup sucanant sugar
   One apple (remove core only)

Mix and boil on low for one hour or more until mixture is thick.

DOUGH:

Place into a vitamix the following:

   One half teaspoon vanilla
   One and a half cups almond butter
   One half teaspoon Biosalt
   One teaspoon rosewater or water
   One cup maple syrup

Mix and add in another bowl, with two cups sifted whole wheat pastry flour.

May add more when needed.

Roll into balls and press into round cookie cutter (2 X 2 inches). Cookies should look like a small pie.

Place on trays lined with parchment paper or a cookie mat, and put into oven.

Bake 5 minutes at 375 degrees.

Then place filling on top cookie and return to oven for 5 more minutes.

This Recipe requires two trays.

Notes: _____

_____

_____

Recipe 322

WALNUT DOME COOKIE

In a large bowl, mix all the following:

> Two cups walnuts (chopped)
> Three cups sucanant sugar
> Four teaspoons vanilla or four teaspoons water
> Three cups maple syrup
> One teaspoon Biosalt
> Three cups almond butter
> Six cups whole wheat pastry flour (sifted)

Mix:

Roll into balls, roll in bowl and coat with coconut flour.

Place on trays lined with parchment paper or cookie mat.

Bake 350 degrees for 20 minutes

Helpful Hints:

Dough will be very thick -- stir then place bowl into microwave oven for 3 minutes and mix.

Notes: _____

_____

_____

Recipe 323

ALMOND DOME COOKIE

In a large bowl, mix all the following:

    Two cups roasted chopped almonds

    Three cups sucanant sugar

    Four teaspoons vanilla or four teaspoons water

    Three cups maple syrup

    One teaspoon Biosalt

    Six cups whole wheat pastry flour (sifted)

    Three cups almond butter

Mix:

Roll into balls one inch by one inch.

Then roll in bowl coconut flour.

Place on trays lined with parchment paper or cookie mat.

Bake 350 degrees for 20 minutes

Helpful Hints:

Dough will be very thick -- stir and place bowl into microwave oven for 3 minutes and mix.

Notes: _____

                _____

Recipe 324 _____

PECAN DOME COOKIE

In a large bowl, mix all the following:

    Two cups pecans chopped
    Three cups Sucanant sugar
    Four teaspoons vanilla or four teaspoons water
    Three cups maple syrup
    One teaspoon Biosalt
    Six cups whole wheat pastry flour (sifted)
    Three cups almond butter

Mix and roll into balls one inch by one inch.

Then roll in bowl coconut flour.

Place on trays lined with parchment paper or cookie mat.

Bake 350 degrees for 20 minutes

Helpful Hints:

Dough will be very thick -- stir and place bowl into microwave oven for 3 minutes and mix.

Notes: _____

           _____

           _____

Recipe 325

CAROB DOME COOKIE

In a large bowl:

Mix all the following:

Two tablespoons carob
Three cups sucanant sugar
Four teaspoons vanilla or four teaspoons water
Two cups walnuts
Three cups maple syrup
One teaspoon Biosalt
Six cups whole wheat pastry flour (sifted)
Three cups almond butter

Mix and roll into balls one inch by one inch.

Then roll in a bowl with coconut flour.

Place on trays lined with parchment paper or cookie mat.

Bake 350 degrees for 20 minutes

Helpful Hints:

Dough will be very thick -- stir and place bowl into microwave oven for 3 minutes and mix.

Notes: _____

_____

_____

Recipe 326

ROMA   DOME COOKIE

In a large bowl, mix all the following:

    Two tablespoons roma
    Three cups sucanant sugar
    Two cups walnuts (chopped)
    One teaspoon Biosalt
    Six cups whole wheat pastry flour (sifted)
    Three cups almond butter

Mix:

Roll into balls the size one inch by one inch.

Then roll in a bowl with coconut flour.

Place on trays lined with parchment paper or cookie mat.

Bake 350 degrees for 20 minutes

Helpful Hints:

Dough will be very thick -- stir and place bowl into microwave oven for 3 minutes and mix

Notes: _____

            _____

            _____

Recipe 327

COFFEE CUP COOKIE

FILLING:

Mix the day before:

Place the following in a vitamix:

> Eight cups sucanant sugar
> Make into powder / then add into a large bowl with:
> One cup soymilk
> Two tablespoons cinnamon
> Two tablespoons Roma
> Eight tablespoons almond butter
> Four tablespoons whole wheat pastry flour
> Six cups walnuts (ground)

Mix and place in refrigerator covered. When ready to use place into microwave oven to soften mixture.

Mix the dough, the day before:

Place into a vitamix the following:

> Three cups maple syrup
> One teaspoon Biosalt
> One teaspoon vanilla
> Two teaspoons water
> Three cups almond butter

Pour into a large bowl mix and add:

Four cups whole wheat pastry flour (sifted)

Place into refrigerator covered. The next day roll dough thin and cut using a round cookie cutter two and a half by 2 and a half or 4 x 4 or both. Can place directly into muffin pans. Do not press dough -- will stick to sides. Then add one to two

tablespoons filling inside cups with one teaspoon to one tablespoon chopped walnuts on top.

Bake 350 degrees for 15 -- 20 minutes.

Makes four and a half to five dozen

Helpful Hints:

Dough will be very thick -- stir and place bowl into microwave oven for 3 minutes and mix

Notes: _____

_____

_____

Recipe 328

RAISIN CUP COOKIE

FILLING:

Mix the day before:

In a vitamix all the following:

One apple (remove core only)

One teaspoon vanilla

One fourth teaspoon Biosalt

Five cups clean raisins -- let drain for one hour

Mix and place in refrigerator covered.

When ready to use place into microwave oven to soften mixture.

The Dough:

Mix the day before.

Place into a vitamix the following:

Three cups maple syrup

One teaspoon Biosalt

One teaspoon vanilla

Two teaspoons water

Three cups almond butter

Mix and pour into a large bowl and add:

Four cups whole wheat pastry flour (sifted)

Place into refrigerator covered. The next day roll dough thin and cut using a round cookie cutter two and a half by two and a half or 4 x 4 or both. Can place directly into muffin pans. Do not press dough -- will stick to sides. Then add one to two

tablespoons filling inside cups with one teaspoon to one tablespoon chopped walnuts on top.

Bake 350 degrees for 15 -- 20 minutes.

Makes four and a half to five dozen

Helpful Hints:

Dough will be very thick -- stir and place bowl into microwave oven for 3 minutes and mix

Notes: _____

_____

_____

Recipe 329

WALNUT CUP COOKIE

FILLING:

Mix the day before:

In a bowl, mix the following:

    Two cups tofu
    Four teaspoons vanilla
    Eight cups walnuts (chopped)
    Four cups sucanant sugar
    Two cups almond butter

Mix and place in refrigerator covered.

When ready to use place into microwave oven to soften mixture.

The Dough:

Mix the day before.

Place into a vitamix the following:

    Three cups maple syrup
    One teaspoon Biosalt
    One teaspoon vanilla
    Two teaspoons water
    Three cups almond butter

Pour into a large bowl and add:

Four cups whole wheat pastry flour (sifted)

Place into refrigerator covered. The next day roll dough thin and cut using a round cookie cutter two and a half by two and a half or 4 x 4 or both. Can place directly into muffin pans. Do not press dough -- will stick to sides. Then add one to two

tablespoons filling inside cups with one teaspoon to one tablespoon chopped walnuts on top.

Bake 350 degrees   for 15 -- 20 minutes.

Makes four and a half to 5 dozen.

Helpful Hints:

Dough will be very thick -- stir and place bowl into microwave oven for 3 minutes and mix.

Notes: _____

‎   _____

‎   _____

Recipe 330

POCKET PIZZA No. 4

For wrap, see Recipe # 274

The Sauce:

Place all the following into a large pan:

> One can olives cut each into one half
> Two onions cut small
> Two bell peppers cut small
> Two carrots shredded
> One stalk celery cut small
> Four cloves garlic cut small
> Two tablespoons Biosalt
> Two teaspoons chili powder
> Two tablespoons maple syrup
> One tablespoon marjoram
> Eleven tomatoes cut small

Then place 11 more tomatoes into vitamix. Do not add any water.

Pour into above pan, Boil for two hours on low.

Pasta:

Pasta - can be any shape - (small.)

Boil per bag instructions after pasta is cooked-- mix with enough sauce to cover.

Stuff into wrap.

Bake 350 degrees for 10 minutes

Let cool. Can freeze extra

Notes: _____

_____

_____

Recipe 331 _____

POCKET PIZZA No. 2

For wrap, see Recipe # 274

Place all the following into a large pan:

> One onion cut small
> One can olives cut each into one half
> Two bell peppers cut small
> Two carrots shredded
> One stalk celery cut small
> Two tablespoons oregano
> Two tablespoons Italian seasoning
> Four cloves garlic cut small
> Two teaspoons Biosalt
> One half teaspoon marjoram

Then place 22 tomatoes or 22 cups into vitamix. Do not add any water.

Pour into above pan, Boil for 2 hours on low.

Pasta:

Pasta - can be any shape - small.

Boil per bag instructions after pasta is cooked-- mix with enough sauce to cover.

Stuff into wrap.

Bake 350 degrees for 10 minutes

Let cool. Can freeze extra.

Notes: _____

_____

_____

Recipe 332

POCKET PIZZA No. 3

For wrap, see Recipe # 274

The Sauce:

Place all the following into a large pan:

>   One onion cut small
>   Two bell peppers cut small
>   One carrot shredded
>   One stalk celery cut small
>   Four teaspoons Italian seasoning
>   Four cloves garlic cut small
>   Two tablespoons Biosalt
>   Two teaspoons basil
>   One tablespoon maple syrup
>   Two teaspoons dill
>   Two teaspoons cumin

Then place 22 tomatoes or 22 cups into vitamix. Do not add any water.

Pour into above pan, Boil for two hours on low.

Pasta:

Pasta - can be any shape - (small.)

Boil per bag instructions after pasta is cooked-- mix with enough sauce to cover.

Stuff into wrap.

Bake 350 degrees for 10 minutes

Let cool. Can freeze extra.

Notes: _____

_____

_____

Recipe 333—————————————————————

POCKET PIZZA No. 1

For wrap, see Recipe # 274

Sauce:

Place all the following into a large pan:

> Eleven tomatoes cut small
> Two onions cut small
> Eight cloves garlic cut small
> One can olives cut each into one half
> One fourth cup paprika
> One tablespoon Biosalt
> One tablespoon maple syrup
> Two tablespoons parsley
> One fourth cup chili powder

Place into vitamix:

Eleven more tomatoes do not add any water.

Then place into above pan.

Boil for two hours on low. Sauce must be thick.

Pasta - can be any shape - small.

Boil per bag instructions after pasta is cooked-- add enough sauce to cover.

Stuff into wrap.

Bake 350 degrees for 10 minutes

Let cool. Can freeze extra.

Notes: _____

_____

_____

Recipe 334

BRAZIL NUT CARMEL CANDY

Place the following into a vitamix for five minutes.

One half cup soymilk

Two teaspoons vanilla
One and one half cups sucanant sugar
One cup maple syrup
One teaspoon Biosalt
One large or two small apples (remove core only)

Then pour into a medium size pan. And boil on warm for 50 - 60 minutes, stir occasionally and prepare dish below:

Line a glass dish 8 X 8 inch with parchment paper and add:

One cup chopped Brazil nuts inside dish and set aside.

Start freezer test 45 minutes into boiling.

Freezer test:

Place in a small dish one spoon the above mixture and place dish in freezer for one minute.

Mixture should be harder at 50 minutes into boiling.

Repeat freezer test at 55 minutes, mixture will be even harder.

At 60 minutes, mixture should be complete.

Pour mixture into glass dish 8 X 8 inch and Place in refrigerator uncovered, for 24 hours.

The next day cut into bite size squares and wrap in wax paper. Store in plastic bag and place in refrigerator.

Notes: _____

_____

_____

Recipe 335

HAVANERO BAKED RICE

The night before soak:

    Five cups water
    Four cups rice

In a baking dish with lid. Set aside.

The next day place into a vitamix all the following:

    One half cup lemon juice
    One and a half cups water
    One tablespoon chili powder
    One tablespoon paprika
    One teaspoon Biosalt
    4 - 6 Havaneros

Then pour into glass dish and mix.

Bake 250 degrees in oven for two hours. All water must be gone.

Let cool with lid on dish.

Place in six ounce cups. Freeze extra.

Notes: _____

_____

_____

*Recipe 336*_____

MACADAMA CARMEL CANDY

Place the following into a vitamix for five minutes.

> One half cup soymilk
> Two teaspoons vanilla
> One and one half cups sucanant sugar
> One teaspoon Biosalt
> One large or two small apples (remove core only)

Then pour into a medium size pan. And boil on warm for 50 - 60 minutes, stir occasionally and prepare dish below:

Line a glass dish 8 X 8 inch with parchment paper and add:

> One cup chopped macadamia nuts inside dish and set aside.

Start freezer test 45 minutes into boiling.

Freezer test:

Place in a small dish one spoon the above mixture and place dish in freezer for one minute.

Mixture should be harder at 50 minutes into boiling.

Repeat freezer test at 55 minutes, mixture will be even harder.

At 60 minutes, mixture should be complete. Pour mixture into glass dish 8 X 8 inch and

Place in refrigerator uncovered, for 24 hours.

The next day cut into bite size squares and wrap in wax paper. Store in plastic bag and place in refrigerator.

Notes: _____

_____

_____

Recipe 337————————————————————

CINNAMON CARMEL CANDY

Place the following into a vitamix for five minutes.

    One tablespoon cinnamon
    Two teaspoons vanilla
    One half cup sucanant sugar
    One cup maple syrup
    One teaspoon Biosalt
    One large or two small apples (remove core only)

Then pour into a medium size pan. And boil on warm for 50 - 60 minutes, stir occasionally and prepare dish below:

Line a glass dish 8 X 8 inch with parchment paper and add:

    One cup chopped walnuts inside dish and set aside.

Start freezer test 45 minutes into boiling.

Freezer test:

Place in a small dish one spoon the above mixture and place dish in freezer for one minute.

Mixture should be harder at 50 minutes into boiling.

Repeat freezer test at 55 minutes, mixture will be even harder.

At 60 minutes, mixture should be complete. Pour mixture into glass dish 8 X 8 inch and Place in refrigerator uncovered, for 24 hours.

The next day cut into bite size squares and wrap in wax paper. Store in plastic bag and place in refrigerator.

Notes: _____

_____

_____

Recipe 338

WALNUT CARMEL CANDY

Place the following into a vitamix for five minutes.

> One half cup soymilk
> Two teaspoons vanilla
> One half cup sucanant sugar
> One cup maple syrup
> One teaspoon Biosalt
> One large or two small apples (remove core only)

Then pour into a medium size pan. And boil on warm for 50 - 60 minutes, stir occasionally and prepare dish below:

Line a glass dish 8 X 8 inch with parchment paper and add:

> One cup chopped walnuts inside dish and set aside.

Start freezer test 45 minutes into boiling.

Freezer test:

Place in a small dish one spoon the above mixture and place dish in freezer for one minute.

Mixture should be harder at 50 minutes into boiling. Repeat freezer test at 55 minutes, mixture will be even harder

At 60 minutes, mixture should be complete. Pour mixture into glass dish 8 X 8 inch and Place in refrigerator uncovered, for 24 hours.

The next day cut into bite size squares and wrap in wax paper. Store in plastic bag and place in refrigerator.

Notes: _____

_____

_____

Recipe 339

COCONUT CARMEL CANDY

Place the following into a vitamix for five minutes.

    One half cup soymilk
    Two teaspoons vanilla
    One half cup sucanant sugar
    One cup maple syrup
    One teaspoon Biosalt
    One large or two small apples (remove core only)

Then pour into a medium size pan. And boil on warm for 50 - 60 minutes, stir occasionally and prepare dish below:

Line a glass dish 8 X 8 inch with parchment paper and add:

    One cup coconut flour inside dish and set aside.

Start freezer test 45 minutes into boiling.

Freezer test:

Place in a small dish one spoon the above mixture and place dish in freezer for one minute.

Mixture should be harder at 50 minutes into boiling.

Repeat freezer test at 55 minutes, mixture will be even harder.

At 60 minutes, mixture should be complete. Pour mixture into glass dish 8 X 8 inch and Place in refrigerator uncovered, for 24 hours.

he next day cut into bite size squares and wrap in wax paper. Store in plastic bag and place in refrigerator.

Notes: _____

_____

_____

Recipe 340

PECAN CARMEL CANDY

Place the following into a vitamix for five minutes.

> One half cup soymilk
> Two teaspoons vanilla
> One half cup sucanant sugar
> One cup maple syrup
> One teaspoon Biosalt
> One large or two small apples (remove core only)

Then pour into a medium size pan. And boil on warm for 50 - 60 minutes, stir occasionally and prepare dish below:

Line a glass dish 8 X 8 inch with parchment paper and add:

> One cup chopped pecans inside dish and set aside.

Start freezer test 45 minutes into boiling.

Freezer test:

Place in a small dish one spoon the above mixture and place dish in freezer for one minute.

Mixture should be harder at 50 minutes into boiling, repeat freezer test at 55 minutes, mixture will be even harder.

At 60 minutes, mixture should be complete. Pour mixture into glass dish 8 X 8 inch and Place in refrigerator uncovered, for 24 hours.

The next day cut into bite size squares and wrap in wax paper. Store in plastic bag and place in refrigerator.

Notes: _____

_____

_____

Recipe 341

PISTACHIO CARMEL CANDY

Place the following into a vitamix for five minutes.

> One half cup soymilk
> Two teaspoons vanilla
> One half cup sucanant sugar
> One cup maple syrup
> One teaspoon Biosalt
> One large or two small apples (remove core only)

Then pour into a medium size pan. And boil on warm for 50 - 60 minutes, stir occasionally and prepare dish below:

Line a glass dish 8 X 8 inch with parchment paper and add:

> One cup Pistachio nuts (chopped)   inside dish and set aside.

Start freezer test 45 minutes into boiling.

Freezer test:

Place in a small dish one spoon the above mixture and place dish in freezer for one minute.

Mixture should be harder at 50 minutes into boiling, repeat freezer test at 55 minutes, mixture will be even harder.

At 60 minutes, mixture should be complete. Pour mixture into glass dish 8 X 8 inch and Place in refrigerator uncovered, for 24 hours.

The next day cut into bite size squares and wrap in wax paper. Store in plastic bag and place in refrigerator.

Notes: _____

_____

_____

Ingredients to Avoid

Bha-butylated bht hydroytolune

Black Strap Molasses

Caffeine

Calcium Sulfate

Carmel

Carrageen

Disodium Sulfite

Distilled water - (do not use- no minerals)

Edtacalcium disodium

Ethylenediamine

Letracetate

Gum Arabic

Cellulose chatti karaya

Gypsum

Hydroylated lecithin

Monocalcium   Satisfactory Phosphate

Hydrolyzed protein

Lactic Acid

Magnesium chlorate

Maltodextrim - white sugar

Magnesium Sterate

Modified food starch

Mono+dislycerides

Mono sodium glutamate

M S G

Multol dextrin

Natural flavor

Nisarl

Non hydroxylated Lecithin

Phosforic acid

Popylgallate

Propylene Glycolalginate

Polysorbate 60, 65, 80
Red Dye 40 - Allura Red AC
Stearic Acid
Sodium Saccharin
Sodium Alginate
Sodium Benzoate
Sodium Bicarbonate
Sodium Chloride
Sodium Erythrobate
Sulfur Dioxide
Sugar black paperbicarbonate of soda
Tragacanth Xanthan
Torutein
Vinegar
Yeast flakes

Recipe LIST

1. BAKED POTATO
2. SALADS
3. PASTA
4. PASTA SAUCE - TOMATO SAUCE
5. BROWN RICE
6. TEXAN RICE
7. BELL PEPPER RICE
8. TOSTADAS
9. POPCORN
10. HOT SAUCE
11. CINDY HUCK BEANS FOR BURRITOS
12. TODD NEUMILLER CHINESE SOUP
13. ALMOND BUTTER
14. PIZZA SAUCE
15. PIZZA DOUGH (FOR PIES)
16. WAFFLES
17. TAMALE CASSEROLE
18. MAPLE SYRUP CAKE
19. PAN - FRIED NOODLES
20. FRUIT ICING
21. CAROB BAKED ALASKA
22. VANILLA CAKE
23. CAROB GLAZE
24. MAPLE OATMEAL CAKE
25. CLOVE COOKIES
26. DONALD W. HUCK COCONUT COOKIES

27. CAROB ROMA OATMEAL COOKIES

28. DEEP - DISH PIZZA

29. COCONUT OATMEAL CAROB ROMA COOKIES

30. COCONUT OATMEAL COOKIES

31. CAROB ROMA COCONUT OATMEAL WHOLE-WHEAT PASTRY FLOUR COOKIES

32. COCONUT OATMEAL WHOLE WHEAT PASTRY FLOUR COOKIES

33. STUFFED BELL PAPPERS

34. MAPLE SYRUP COOKIES

35. CAROB COOKIES

36. CAROB BROWN CAKE

37. ANY FRUIT COOKIES (PEACH, CHERRY, APRICOT)

38. SPECIAL PIE CRUST

39. PUMPKIN PIE

40. PARVIN MALEK CAROB PIE

41. ALMOND BUTTER COOKIES 2

42. CAROB FILLING

43. EVELYN ANN MENZIE OLD-FASHIONED GLAZE

44. PINEAPPLE PIE

45. BUTTER COOKIES

46. SUCANANT COOKIES

47. INEZ A. MENZIE COCONUT COOKIES

48. TURNOVERS

49. GOLDEN MACAROONS

50. ORIENTAL CRUNCH

51. PINEAPPLE CANDY

52. CAROB DOUGHNUTS

53. LEMON DOUGHNUTS

54. GRAIN PIZZA

55. CORNMEAL PIZZA

56. CAROB BROWNIES

57. ROBERT E MENZIE WALNUT PIE

58. APRICOT COCONUT WALNUT SQUARES

59. PISTACHIO SCONES

60. EGG ROLLS

61. ROASTED SALTED NUTS

62. FUDGE CUP COOKIE

63. FUDGE SAUCE

64. PINEAPPLE COOKIES

65. TAMALE BEAN PIE

66. NUT PIE

67. DATE WALNUT COOKIES

68. CARAMELIZED GINGER HAZELNUT TART

69. PAPAYA COOKIES

70. CAJUN MIXED NUTS

71. TACO SALAD SHELLS

72. FOR CAKE-WEDDING STYLE CAKE

73. SPANISH MILLET CASSEROLE

74. ENCHILADAS

75. CAROB PIE

76. NUT BUTTER BALLS

77. SHARAREH SHABAFROOZ GARLIC BREAD SPREAD/BUTTER

78. GLAZED CARROT CAKE

79. WAFFLES WITH CASHEWS AND OATMEAL

80. LEMON PINEAPPLE PIE

81. CORN BREAD

82. MATTHEW F. MOONEY ROAST FOR ANY HOLIDAY

83. SPICE DOUGHNUTS

84. SPANISH RICE

85. PINEAPPLE SANDWICH COOKIE

86. CAROB CUP COOKIE

87. ANY FRUIT CUP COOKIE

88. SETAREH TAIS CAKE

89. CAROB DATE PISTACHIO PASTRY

90. FRUIT CAKE COOKIE

91. BAKED MILLET

92. BISCOTTI

93. MULTIGRAIN CRACKERS

94. POT PIE

95. BASIC COOKIE WITH FROSTING

96. TACO SHELLS

97. ANY FRUIT PASTRY

98. PINEAPPLE FROSTING

99. PINEAPPLE UPSIDE DOWN CAKE

100. HOT BEANS FOR BURRITOS

101. APRICOT PIE

102. APPLE PIE

103. PLUM PIE

104. PIZZA SAUCE NO. 3

105. PIZZA SAUCE NO. 1

106. COFFEE MUFFINS

107. GLORIA DUGGINS PECAN CANDY

108. PETER P. PANAGOPOULOS ALMOND FUDGE

109. PETE/ROSA CERRILLO CINNAMON WALNUT CANDY

110. SUGARED NUTS

111. PAPAYA CANDY

112. CAROB CAKE

113. THELMA MAIN HAZELNUT FUDGE

114. WHEAT CORNMEAL PIZZA

115. MARGARET/HARVEY BINDER PECAN FUDGE

116. MICHAEL F. MOONEY PECAN ROMA CAROB CANDY

117. BELLE HUCK WALNUT FUDGE

118. SAUCE FOR INSIDE CINNAMON ROLLS

119. NECTARINE PIE

120. COOKIES/CAROB PLAIN OR ROMA

121. CAROB BARS

122. SPICE BUTTER COOKIES

123. OAT CRACKERS

124. CINNAMON SUGAR DOUGHNUT TOPPING

125. JELLY DOUGHNUT FILLING

126. STRUDEL DOUGH

127. DATE CUP COOKIE

128. ITALIAN SAUCE

129. LASAGNA

130. BOB PANAGOPOULOS PIZZA SAUCE NO. 2

131. CUBAN BLACK BEANS IN RICE

132. BLACK BEANS

133. LIGHT FUDGE

134. DARK FUDGE

135. PIGEON BEANS

136. XENIA PANAGOPOULOS PIGEON RICE

137. ALEXANDRA PANAGOPOULOS SWEET AND SOUR SAUCE NO. 1

138. INEZ SPEIDELL SWEET AND SOUR SAUCE NO. 2

139. VERY VERY HOT SAUCE

140. LENTILS

141. SHRIMP SAUCE

142. GABRIEL CERRILLO ALMOND CAROB CANDY

143. CAROB ROMA CANDY

144. WALNUT CINNAMON CLUSTERS

145. TAMARA NEUMILLER SPANISH PASTA

146. CHINESE RICE

147. CHILI BEANS

148. TAMALES

149. VEGETABLE SOUP

150. CAROB ROMA COOKIES

151. RAY AND LINDA PANAGOPOULOS SUNFLOWER COCONUT WAFFLES

152. WAFFLES OATMEAL AND ALMONDS

153. RHI CAROB AND ROMA OATMEAL WWP NUTLESS COOKIE

154. HOT SAUCE

155. RED BEANS FOR TOP OF RICE

156. CORN MEAL WAFFLES

157. TAGLIATELLE SAUCE

158. ALMOND BUTTER COOKIES

159. MAPLE SYRUP FROSTING

160. ORANGE GLAZE

161. RYE PANCAKES

162. PANCAKES

163. BLUEBERRY TOPPING

164. ROMA ICE CREAM

165. LEMON ICE CREAM

166. ORANGE DATE SYRUP

167. CAROB FUDGE SAUCE

168. COCONUT LIME FROSTING

169. CREAMY FROSTING

197. COCONUT CAKE

198. PUMPKIN COOKIES

199. MARSELLAS PANAGOPOULOS BRAZIL NUT ICE CREAM

200. TAHEREH MALEK PUMPKIN ICE CREAM

201. BAKED BROWN RICE

202. GINGER CANDY

203. SANDY MOONEY COFFEE CAKE

204. PAPAYA WALNUT COOKIES

205. LEMON CARROT COOKIES

206. CAROB SANDWICH COOKIES

207. DAISY FROSTING

208. BLACK-EYED PEAS

209. ALMOND BUTTER FROSTING

210. CRUNCH TOPPING FOR ANY BAKED PIE

211. CHERI GILBERT COOKED CAROB GLAZE

212. SUCANANT SUGAR GLAZE

213. ROMA CREAM FROSTING

214. LEMON FILLING

215. BAR-B-QUE SAUCE

216. TOFU FROSTING

217. SWEET SUGAR ICING

218. BLACK EYED IN RICE

219. SOY MILK CORNBREAD

220. OATMEAL ALMOND COOKIE

221. SPICED CUPCAKES

222. DATE OATMEAL COOKIE

223. ORANGE COCONUT COOKIE

224. DATE COOKIE BAR

225. APRICOT COOKIE BAR

226. GINGER PANCAKES

227. LEMON PASTRY

228. LEMON SUGAR COOKIES

229. DATE BROWNIES

230. ORIGINAL SALT WATER TAFFY

231. AURA VICTORIA HUCK PEPPERMINT SALT WATER TAFFY

232. LEMON SALT WATER TAFFY

233. VANILLA SALT WATER TAFFY

234. ORANGE SALT WATER TAFFY

235. JACK PANAGOPOULOS ROMA SALT WATER TAFFY

236. ADRIANA CERRILLO PECAN SALT WATER TAFFY

237. ELMER LYLE MENZIE ALMOND SALT WATER TAFFY

238. ASHLEY SPEIDELL WALNUT SALT WATER TAFFY

239. ROSS H. MENZIE CAROB SALT WATER TAFFY

240. COCONUT SALT WATER TAFFY

241. CINAMMON SALT WATER TAFFY

242. GINGER SALT WATER TAFFY

243. GENE KOENIG ENGLISH TOFFEE CANDY

244. LUCILLE GILBERT LEMON CHEESECAKE

245. ORANGE CHEESECAKE

246. ASHER MICHAEL NEUMILLER CAROB CHEESECAKE

247. ALLIE NICOLE BLUMA NEUMILLER CAROB CAKE

248. DR. EDE VANILLA SUGAR CAKE

249. WALNUT SQUARE COOKIES

250. TARA SHABAFROOZ PECAN SQUARE COOKIES

251. ALMOND SQUARE COOKIES

252. MARGRET ANN MENZIE PECAN ROPE COOKIES

253. MASSOOD SHABAFROOZ WALNUT ROPE COOKIES

254. ALMOND ROPE COOKIES

283. POCKET PIZZA 4

284. POCKET PIZZA 2

285. POCKET DATE PASTRY

286. POCKET PLUM PASTRY

287. PLUM CREAM PIE

288. POCKET CAROB PASTRY

289. POCKET ROMA PASTRY

290. POCKET WALNUT PASTRY

291. POCKET APRICOT PASTRY

292. POCKET CHERRY PASTRY

293. POCKET PEACH PASTRY

294. POCKET PINEAPPLE - LEMON PASTRY

295. POCKET PUMPKIN PASTRY

296. POCKET APPLE PASTRY

297. POCKET EGG ROLLS

298. POCKET BEAN BURRITO

299. APRICOT CREAM PIE

300. VERA WALDSCHMIDT CHERRY CREAM PIE

301. PEACH CREAM PIE

302. APPLE CREAM PIE

303. TAHEREH TAHERIAN   HAVANERO HOT SAUCE

304. SHAHNAZ SHAINEE HOT AND SPICY PINTO BEANS

305. PAYAM MALEK ZADEH CAROB WHEAT COOKIES

306. RAISIN ICE CREAM

307. TOMATO CASSEROLE

308. RAISIN FACE COOKIE

309. DATE FACE COOKIE

310. PINEAPPLE COCONUT SQUARES

311. ORANGE PINEAPPLE ICE CREAM

312. LEMON PINEAPPLE ICE CREAM

313. ROMA FACE COOKIE

314. CAROB FACE COOKIE

315. PUMPKIN FACE COOKIE

316. PINEAPPLE FACE COOKIE

317. APPLE FACE COOKIE

318. PEACH FACE COOKIE

319. APRICOT FACE COOKIE

320. PLUM FACE COOKIE

321. CHERRY FACE COOKIE

322. WALNUT DOME COOKIES

323. ALMOND DOME COOKIES

324. PECAN DOME COOKIES

325. CAROB DOME COOKIES

326. ROMA DOME COOKIES

327. COFFEE CUP COOKIE

328. RAISIN CUP COOKIE

329. WALNUT CUP COOKIE

330. POCKET PASTA NO. 4

331. POCKET PASTA NO. 2

332. POCKET PASTA NO. 3

333. POCKET PASTA NO. 1

334. BRAZIL NUT CARMEL CANDY

335. HAVANERO BAKED RICE

336. MACADAMA CARMEL CANDY

337. CINNAMON CARMEL CANDY

338. WALNUT CARMEL CANDY

339. COCONUT CARMEL CANDY

340. PECAN CARMEL CANDY

341. PISTACHIO CARMEL CANDY

342. HAZEL NUT CARMEL CANDY

343. CASHEW CARMEL CANDY

344. ROASTED ALMOND CARMEL CANDY

345. LEMON CARMEL CANDY

346. ORANGE CARMEL CANDY

347. CAROB CARMEL CANDY

348. ROMA CARMEL CANDY

349. PEPPERMINT CARMEL CANDY

350. GINGER CARMEL CANDY

351. HERBS & GARLIC BAKED RICE

352. WALNUT & ALMOND FROSTING

353. PINEAPPLE & LEMON GLAZE

354. ROMA TOFU COOKIES

355. CAROB TOFU COOKIES

356. CINNAMON TOFU COOKIES

357. RAISIN TOFU COOKIES

358. APRICOT TOFU COOKIES

359. DATE TOFU COOKIES

360. CRANBERRIE TOFU COOKIES

361. SPICE TOFU COOKIES

362. PAPAYA TOFU COOKIES

363. COCONUT TOFU COOKIES

364. LEMON TOFU COOKIES

365. ORANGE TOFU COOKIES

366. PINEAPPLE TOFU COOKIES

367. BLACK BEAN SOUP

368. LEMON COCONUT COOKIES

369. CHERRY SUGAR COOKIES

370. ORANGE SUGAR COOKIES

371. RAISIN SUGAR COOKIES

372. ROMA SUGAR COOKIES

373. APPLE SUGAR COOKIES

374. CAROB SUGAR COOKIES

375. PEPPERMINT SUGAR COOKIES

376. BLUEBERRY SUGAR COOKIE

377. DATE SUGAR COOKIE

378. PINEAPPLE SUGAR COOKIE

379. PLUM SUGAR COOKIE

380. PEACH SUGAR COOKIE

381. APRICOT SUGAR COOKIE

382. NECTURINE SUGAR COOKIE

383. CRANBERRY SUGAR COOKIE

384. PUMPKIN SUGAR COOKIE

385. COCONUT CAROB CARMEL CANDY

386. COCONUT LEMON CARMEL CANDY

387. COCONUT CINNAMON CARMEL CANDY

388. COCONUT ORANGE CARMEL CANDY

389. COCONUT PEPPERMINT CARMEL CANDY

390. COCONUT ROMA CARMEL CANDY

391. COCONUT GINGER CARMEL CANY

392. DATE OATMEAL COOKIE

393. RAISIN OATMEAL COOKIE

394. WALNUT DATE COOKIE

395. WALNUT LEMON COOKIE

396. WALNUT RAISIN COOKIE

397. WALNUT ORANGE COOKIE

398. WALNUT CHERRY COOKIE

399. COCONUT DATE COOKIE

400. COCONUT CHERRY COOKIE

401. COCONUT RAISIN COOKIE

402. ONION DRIED ROASTED NUTS

403. GARLIC DRIED ROASTED NUTS

404. HAVANERO DRIED ROASTED NUTS

405. CAYANE DRIED ROASTED NUTS

406. BLACK BEAN RICE

407. SALTED-HAVANERO DRIED ROASTED NUT MIX

408. MAPLE SYRUP DRIED ROASTED NUTS

409. CAROB MACROONS

410. LEMON MACROONS

411. ROMA MACROONS

412. ORANGE MACROONS

413. PEPPERMINT FROSTING

414. PINEAPPLE-LEMON BAKED ALASKA

415. LEMON BAKED ALASKA

416. ORANGE BAKED ALASKA

417. PEPERMINT BAKED ALASKA

418. VANILLA BAKED ALASKA

419. RED HOT FIRE SAUCE

420. APRICOT ICE CREAM

421. TWICE COOKED HERB POTATO

422. PEPPERMINT MACROONS

423. PEACH ICE CREAM

424. TWICE COOKED SPICY POTATO

425. PLUM MACROONS

426. SPICY GARLIC SPREAD

427. ITALIAN SPREAD

428. WALNUT WAFFLES

429. POPPY SEED WAFFLES

430. PUMPKIN SEED WAFFLES

431. CAROB SUCANAT SUGAR COOKIE

432. ROMA SUCANAT SUGAR COOKIE

433. PEPPERMINT SUCANAT SUGAR COOKIE

434. CINNAMON SUCANAT SUGAR COOKIE

435. GINGER SUCANAT SUGAR COOKIE

436. CAROB SUGARED NUTS

437. ROMA SUGARED NUTS

438. PECAN PIE

439. BLUEBERRY CREAM PIE

440. GRAPE PIE

441. LEMON FROSTING

442. ORANGE   CAKE FROSTING

443. VANILLA CAKE FROSTING

444. PEACH   MAPLE CAKE

445. PLUM   MAPLE CAKE

446. APRICOT MAPLE CAKE

447. PINEAPPLE MAPLE CAKE

448. APPLE MAPLE CAKE

449. CHERRY MAPLE CAKE

450. NECTURINE MAPLE CAKE

451. LEMON MAPLE CAKE

452. ORANGE MAPLE CAKE

453. BLUEBERRY MAPLE CAKE

454. PEAR MAPLE CAKE

455. BLUEBERRY BAKED ALASKA

456. BAR- B- QUE HOT SAUCE

457. PISTACHIO WAFFELS

458. PEACH BAKED ALASKA

459. APRICOT BAKED ALASKA

460. APPLE BAKED ALASKA

461. PLUM BAKED ALASKA

462. NECTURINE BAKED ALASKA

463. GRAPE BAKED ALASKA

464. CHEESE SAUCE FOR BAKED POTATO

465. APPLE ICE CREAM

466. PLUM ICE CREAM

467. GRAPE ICE CREAM

468. PEAR ICE CREAM

469. RHI MAPLE SYRUP COOKIES

470. MAPLE SYRUP BROWNIES

471. CAROB NUGGET CANDY

472. ROMA NUGGET CANDY

473. PEPPERMINT NUGGET CANDY

474. CINNAMON NUGGET CANDY

475. LEMON NUGGET CANDY

476. VANILLA NUGGET CANDY

477. APRICOT NUGGET CANDY

478. ITALIAN DRY ROASTED NUT MIX

479. GARLIC DRY ROASTED PUFF CORN MIX

480. ONION DRY ROASTED PUFF CORN MIX

481. HAVENARO DRY ROASTED PUFF CORN MIX

482. CAYENNE DRY ROASTED PUFF CORN MIX

483. ITALIAN DRY ROASTED PUFF CORN MIX

484. SALTED DRY ROASTED PUFF CORN MIX

485. CAJUN DRY ROASTED PUFF CORN MIX

486. SALTED HAVENARO DRY ROASTED PUFF C ORN MIX

487. PLUM TOFU COOKIES

488 . PEACH TOFU COOKIES

489. NECTARINE TOFU COOKIES

490. SPICY AVACADO DIP

491. ALL PURPOSE GRAVY

492. POTATO AND CABBAGE STEW

493. CAROB PIE CRUST

494. ROMA PIE CRUST

495. COFFEE BAKED PIE

496. CRANBERRY SAUCE

497. GREEN BEANS CASSAROLE

498. QUICK OATMEAL

499. BAKED YAMS

500. SAUTE CORN

501. CINNAMON AND GINGER COOKIES

502. ORANGE NUGGET CANDY

503. POTATO AND CELERY SOUP

504. AVACADO DIP

505. CARROT SOUP

506. PEACH UPSIDE DOWN CREAM CAKE

507. APRICOT UPSIDE DOWN CREAM CAKE

508. NECTARINE UPSIDE DOWN CREAM CAKE

509. CHERRY UPSIDE DOWN CREAM CAKE

510. GRAPE UPSIDE DOWN CREAM CAKE

511. APPLE UPSIDE DOWN CREAM CAKE

512. CINNAMON UPSIDE DOWN CREAM CAKE

513. CAROB UPSIDE DOWN CREAM CAKE

514. PLUM UPSOIDE DOWN CREAM CAKE

515. ROMA UPSIDE DOWN CREAM CAKE

516. PINEAPPLE UPSIDE DOWN CREAM CAKE

517. PEPPERMINT UPSIDE DOWN CREAM CAKE

518. ORANGE UPSIDE DOWN CREAM CAKE

519. LEMON UPSIDE DOWN CREAM CAKE

520. GINGER UPSIDE DOWN CREAM CAKE

521. JAMACIAN RICE

522. LEMON AND OLIVE BASMATI RICE MIX

523. CARROT AND OLIVE BASMATI RICE MIX

524. GARLIC AND ONION SAUTED CORN

525. GREEN JALAPENO RICE MIX

526. ROASTED PISTACHIO CANDY

527. PISTACHIO FUDGE

528. SPICY CORN BREAD

529. RED HOT ROAST

530. CINNAMON WALNUT COOKIES

531. ORANGE BALL COOKIES

532. LEMON BALL COOKIES

533. ORANGE PASTRY

534. CINNAMON MACROONS

535. CINNAMON AND OATMEAL COOKIES

536. RED POTATO CASSEROLE

537. CINNAMON ICE CREAM

538. DATE WALNUT TART

539. WALNUT GINGER COOKIES

540. WALNUT ROMA COOKIES

541. WALNUT CAROB COOKIES

542. SLICE WALNUT COOKIES

543. LEMON AND HERB DRY ROASTED NUT MIX

544. LEMON AND DILL DRY ROASTED NUT MIX

545. LEMON AND SALTED DRY ROASTED NUT MIX

546. SWEET AND SOUR DRY ROASTED NUT MIX

547. LEMON AND CAYANNE DRY ROASTED NUT MIX

548. LEMON AND CAJON DRY ROASTED NUT MIX

549. LEMON AND HAVENERO ROASTED NUT MIX

550. LEMON AND ONION DRY ROASTED NUT MIX

551. LEMON AND GARLIC DRY ROASTED NUT MIX

552. NECTURINE ICE CREAM

553. SPICE ICE CREAM

554. THIN CORN BREAD

555. NECTURINE CREAM PIE

556. CINNAMON PIE

557. CINNAMON CHEESE CAKE

558. CINNAMON DATE PASTRY

559. CARMELIZED CINNAMON TART

560. CINNAMON CANDY

561. LICORICE ICE CREAM

562. LICORICE FROSTING

563. LICORICE BAKED ALASKA

564. LICORICE CHEESE CAKE

565. LICORICE TOFFEE COOKIES

566. LICORICE FUDGE

567. LICORICE SALT WATER TOFFEE

568. LICORICE COCONUT CARMELS

569. LICORICE CANDY

570. LICORICE COCONUT COOKIES

571. LICORICE MACROONS

572. HAVANERO RICE

573. MARTIN MASSOOD TAIS LICORICE SANDWICH COOKIES

574. CINNAMON SANDWICH COOKIES

575. CORN ON THE COB

576. AVA DANIELLE NUEMILLER ORANGE CREAM PIE

577. CINNAMON WALNUT FUDGE

578. WALNUT CRUST FOR ANY PIE

579. GREEN PEAS AND RICE

580. LEMON CREAM PIE

581. COCONUT CREAM PIE

582. PUMPKIN AND APPLE COOKIES

583. SUCANANT FACE COOKIES

584. HAZEL NUT FACE COOKIES

585. HAZEL NUT CAROB COOKIES

586. PISTACHIO FACE COOKIES

587. PISTACHIO AND CASHEW COOKIES

588. PERO SUCANANT COOKIES

589. HAZELNUT SPICE COOKIES

590. CINNAMON WALNUT FACE COOKIES

591. CAROB-COCONUT FACE COOKIES

592. LEMON WALNUT COOKIES

593. ORANGE WALNUT COOKIES

594. ANISE WALNUT COOKIES

595. PEPPERMINT WALNUT COOKIES

596. CAROB COCONUT PIE COOKIES

597. PERO AND HAZELNUT PIE COOKIES

598. CARMELIZED CINNAMON PISTACHIO TART

599. VITAMIX LICORICE MACROONS

600. VITAMIX CINNAMON MACROONS

References

John Robbins

Dr. Ede Koenig

"The Whole Kernal"

PDR, "Physicians Desk Reference"

About the Author

For almost the past ten years understanding health has been very interesting, and I have applied this information to improve my life. I have and will continue to inspire others who want to do the same. I give away thousands of food items yearly and encourage others to share their food. I develop and research food Recipes, adding to my approximate 600 Recipes to date. I have won 55 awards for my cooking, in addition, have written eight books on health and cooking. All books include Recipes, which work in concert with a healthy body. Most of all I continue to maintain a healthy life style and I am an example of what good food and a clean body can accomplish. As I share this information, I hope to show how easy this completely healthy life style is to achieve. These benefits are incredible, and not limited to only a few. I will never go back to a life of pain and suffering and declining health. There is just no legitimate reason to not maintain a healthy life style through good nutrition and avoidance of all drugs.

Science cannot replace nature and cannot fool the body. In the long term, the body will malfunction if not treated properly. I can say for certain that to continue abusing the body and maintaining disease with drugs does not make any sense. Research done on drugs in the United States shows that good health and drugs are not related, but to avoid sickness through proper nutrition will guarantee good health and are closely related.